Guide to Arthrocentesis and Soft Tissue Injection

Bruce Carl Anderson, MD

Clinical Associate Professor of Medicine
Oregon Health Sciences University

Medical Orthopedic Department
Sunnyside Medical Center
Portland, Oregon

D1617324

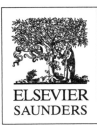

ELSEVIER
SAUNDERS

ELSEVIER
SAUNDERS

The Curtis Center
170 S Independence Mall W 300E
Philadelphia, Pennsylvania 19106

GUIDE TO ARTHROCENTESIS AND SOFT TISSUE INJECTION ISBN 0-4160-2205-8
Copyright © 2005, Elsevier Inc.

NOTICE

Library of Congress Cataloging-in-Publication Data

Anderson, Bruce Carl
    Guide to arthrocentesis and soft tissue injection / Bruce Carl Anderson.
        p. ; cm.
    Includes bibliographical references and index.
    ISBN 1-4160-2205-8 (alk. paper)
    1. Arthrocentesis. 2. Joints—Diseases—Diagnosis. 3. Diagnosis, Differential. I. Title.
    [DNLM: 1. Injections—methods. 2. Joint Diseases—drug therapy. 3. Diagnosis,
Differential. 4. Joint Diseases—diagnosis. 5. Pain—drug therapy. 6. Punctures—methods.
WE 304 A545h 2005]
RC932.A52 2005
616.7′206—dc22   2004061428

Acquisitions Editor: Rolla Couchman
Publishing Services Manager: Frank Polizzano
Project Manager: Lee Ann Draud
Design Coordinator: Karen O'Keefe Owens

Printed in the United States of America.

Last digit is the print number: 9   8   7   6   5   4   3   2   1

Working together to grow
libraries in developing countries
www.elsevier.com | www.bookaid.org | www.sabre.org

ELSEVIER   BOOK AID International   Sabre Foundation

To

Dr. James Cyriax
British Doctor of Medicine and Osteopathy
Father of Medical Orthopedics

Preface

This guide is not all-inclusive by any means. There are as many ways to approach the diagnosis and as many treatments to achieve a successful outcome as there are musculoskeletal conditions. I acknowledge that widespread differences remain in diagnostic testing, injection technique, choice of medication, and physical therapy exercising. This diversity remains simply because the number of scientific studies devoted to the subject of medical orthopedics in the literature is still relatively limited. The purpose of this guide is to serve as a starting point for clinicians interested in expanding their expertise in the diagnosis and treatment of these exceedingly common musculoskeletal conditions and generate enough interest to initiate evidence-based scientific studies.

It is time to discard the notion that injuries to the soft tissues are strictly under the auspices of the department of surgical orthopedics and injuries and inflammations of the joints are strictly under the purview of the department of rheumatology. We need to follow the lead of the British system of medicine (see volumes I and II of James Cyriax's *Textbook of Orthopaedic Medicine*) and incorporate this overlooked area of medicine into the core curricula of residency programs in medicine, family practice, and osteopathy. I hope that this guide and my other major work, *Office Orthopedics for Primary Care*, can serve as a bridge among the departments of rheumatology, orthopedics, neurology, physical medicine, podiatry, and osteopathy and provide the stimulation to greater interest, discussion, and research in the diagnosis and treatment of the conditions that affect the musculoskeletal system.

Bruce Carl Anderson, MD

Acknowledgments

This guide represents the outgrowth of 26 years of postresidency clinical education and experience that would not have been possible without the support and encouragement from many sources. I wish to thank all the members of the Department of Medicine and Surgical Orthopedics at Sunnyside Medical Center, with special thanks to Dr. Ian MacMillan and Linda Onheiber—my extremely capable physician assistant—for their continual support, especially in the early years. I wish to thank all the medical residents of the graduating classes of 2003 and 2004 at the Oregon Health Science University, Legacy Emanuel Hospital and Health Center, the Sisters of Providence, and the Eastmoreland osteopathic teaching hospitals for their constant encouragement, contributions, and critical appraisal of the content of the guide (especially Dr. Amy Chaumeton, Dr. Ali Bahar, Dr. Keith Bachman, and Dr. Amy Simantel). I wish to thank Dr. David N. Gilbert—my Internal Medicine Residency Director—for his stimulation to excellence, his encouragement to examine ever deeper into clinical problems, and his support and inspiration to return to clinical research.

Contents

GENERAL CONCEPTS OF LOCAL MUSCULOSKELETAL INJECTION

PRINCIPLES

Successful management of the conditions affecting the musculoskeletal system requires the combination of the available treatment modalities that specifically arrests the body's exaggerated *inflammatory reaction*, corrects the degree of *mechanical dysfunction*, and acts to prevent *tissue damage*. This includes determining the proper sequencing of the following treatments: (1) **local anesthetic block** to confirm the clinical diagnosis; (2) separate **corticosteroid injection** using a "long-acting" and concentrated derivative to arrest the inflammatory response (undiluted and unmixed with anesthetic and placed anatomically as opposed to trigger point injection); (3) **rest and restricted use** following injection to minimize displacement, lessen the "inflammatory flare reaction," and achieve the optimal anti-inflammatory effect; (4) **adjunctive physical therapy** exercises to recover or enhance lost function; (5) restricted use and long-term physical therapy exercises to **prevent** recurrence; and (6) **orthopedic surgical** referral for advanced cases with loss of function, persistent pain, or tissue damage.

MATERIALS

The following materials are required to perform the procecdures in this manual: (1) iodine and alcohol preps; (2) ethyl chloride topical spray; (3) 1% lidocaine without epinephrine; (4) depot methylprednisolone 80 mg/mL (D80); triamcinolone acetonide 40 mg/mL (K40); tri-iodinated meglumine diatrizoate radiopaque contrast; (5) 3-, 5-, 10-, and 25-mL disposable syringes; (6) $\frac{5}{8}$-inch, 25-gauge; $1\frac{1}{2}$-inch, 22-gauge; $3\frac{1}{2}$-inch, 22-gauge spinal; $1\frac{1}{2}$-inch, 18-gauge needles; (7) a medium size hemostat to facilitate changing syringes; (8) adhesive bandages, 4 × 4 gauze, 1-inch tape, and elastic wrap (Coban); and (9) access to orthopedic braces, splints, and casting.

EXPLANATION AND REASSURANCE

Of the variety of procedures used in clinical medicine, joint and soft tissue injection provokes the greatest degree of anxiety. This exaggerated concern is due to the general fear of needle insertion, the layman's rumors of previous negative experience with injection, and the misconception that side effects of injectable steroids are the same as orally administered steroids. In order to ameliorate these concerns and engender greater patient confidence and trust, the examiner must provide a thorough explanation of the goals of treatment and the details of the procedure. Each patient should be counseled on the following issues: (1) the use of topical anesthesia, (2) the careful use of local anesthesia, (3) the relatively benign side effects of injectable steroids, (4) the need to control inflammation to allow the body to heal more effectively, (5) the importance of combining treatments, and (6) the expected outcome.

"A properly performed injection should cause no more than 1 second of pain when using ethyl chloride freeze spray on the skin and local anesthetic placed over the first tissue plane!"

"There's no question that cortisone causes serious side effects, such as weight gain, 'moon' face, an elevated blood sugar, high blood pressure, and loss of calcium. However, these side effects develop much more commonly with cortisone pills taken by mouth and very uncommonly with injection."

"This is a very small dose of cortisone …. Did you know your body makes 20 to 30 mg of cortisone every day? The cortisone used in injection is only 5% to 10% different than the natural cortisone you produce in your body every day. The dose is so small and so isolated, it rarely interferes with your body's metabolism!"

"Cortisone given by injection is the single most effective treatment of local inflammation! Would you ignore the inflammation of an infected cut?"

"Cortisone injection is but 'one tool' used in treatment. It dramatically reduced pain and inflammation, allowing you to perform your recovery exercises more effectively."

SKIN PREPARATION

The operator should glove for protection. Iodine followed by alcohol scrub is used to prepare the injection site. Injection is contraindicated in the presence of infected skin, chronically inflamed skin, or systemic infection.

ANESTHETIC INJECTION

A separate anesthetic injection is important for the following reasons: (1) to confirm the diagnosis, especially when two conditions exist simultaneously, (2) to exclude a potential complication (rotator cuff tendinitis versus tendon tear), and (3) to avoid dilution of the corticosteroid (anesthetic is placed in several layers, whereas the corticosteroid is injected in a single tissue plane or structure). For example, in the treatment of a dorsal ganglion, anesthetic is injected outside the cyst wall, the viscous fluid is aspirated completely, and corticosteroid is injected undiluted into the drained cyst.

CORTICOSTEROID INJECTION

The concentrated (mg/mL), long-acting corticosteroid derivatives, when injected undiluted into a bursa, joint, or tissue plane, provide the most predictable results. The soluble derivatives do not provide a long enough suppression of inflammation to be as effective.

INJECTION TECHNIQUE AND VOLUME

Once the point of entry has been chosen, the needle is passed gently through the tissues. The syringe should be held with the lightest of touch (as if holding a dart) so that as the needle encounters and penetrates each tissue, the resistance and pressure of each level can be fully appreciated (fat has the least tissue resistance and bone the greatest, with muscle, synovial membrane, ligament, and tendon intermediate!). If the patient experiences discomfort, the operator should pause, inject anesthetic, partly withdraw the needle, and redirect the needle away from the painful site. All injections of anesthetic or corticosteroid should be performed slowly with the least volume to avoid tissue disruption.

PRECAUTIONS

At the completion of the injection, firm pressure should be immediately applied. The patient must avoid all known aggravations for the first **3 days** (to protect the injection site) and to limit these for **30 days.** In selected cases (Achilles tendinitis, for example), fixed immobilization may be necessary. Any restrictions that the patient has placed upon him- or herself for the past 30 days should be continued for 4 weeks, until the full effect of the medication has been realized!

SIDE EFFECTS

The side effects from injectable steroids are limited to local reactions. Systemic effects as seen with oral steroids are uncommon. All patients must be warned about (1) the 30% chance of soreness or pain after the injection (2 to 3 days; ice; acetaminophen), (2) the 10% risk of an inflammatory flare reaction (2 to 3 days; ice; narcotics), (3) the 30% chance of fat or skin atrophy (only superficial injections with 90% reverting back to normal in 6 to 12 months), (4) the necessity of reevaluation if redness, swelling, and pain persist beyond 3 to 4 days (chance of infection 1:10,000 or less), and (5) signs of a more complicated condition.

PHYSICAL THERAPY EXERCISES

Local injection must be followed by physical therapy recovery exercises to optimize the overall outcome of treatment. The appropriate exercises are usually begun on the fourth day and gradually increased over the next 3 to 4 weeks. All recommended times of rest, restriction of use, and recovery exercises are based on average responses. Individual cases can be treated with specific recommendations based on response and tolerance.

Chapter 1

NECK

THE DIFFERENTIAL DIAGNOSIS OF NECK PAIN

DIAGNOSES	CONFIRMATIONS
Cervical strain (most common diagnosis)	
Stress	Socioeconomic or psychological issues
Whiplash and related injuries	Motor vehicle accident or head and neck trauma
Dorsokyphotic posture	Typical posture seen in the elderly or in patients with depression
Fibromyalgia	Confirmation by examination: multiple trigger points; normal laboratory results
Osteoarthritis of the neck	Radiographs: cervical series (lateral view)
"Reactive cervical strain"	The underlying spinal column or cord is threatened
Radiculopathy	Neurologic testing
Vertebral body fracture	Bone scan or magnetic resonance imaging (MRI)
Spinal cord injury or tumor	MRI
Cervical radiculopathy	
Foraminal encroachment	Radiographs: cervical spine (oblique views); electromyogram (EMG)
Herniated nucleus pulposus	MRI
Cervical rib	Radiographs: cervical series (anteroposterior view)
Thoracic outlet syndrome	Nerve conduction velocity (NCV)/EMG
Epidural process	MRI
Greater occipital neuritis	
Referred pain	
Coronary arteries	Electrocardiogram, creatine phosphokinase, angiogram
Takayasu's arteritis	Erythrocyte sedimentation rate (ESR), angiogram
Thoracic aortic aneurysm	Chest radiograph
Thyroid disease	Thyroid-stimulating hormone, T4, ESR, thyroid scan

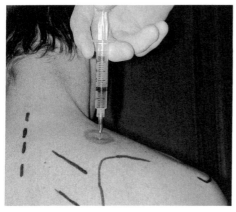

Enter the upper trapezius muscle at the point of maximum tenderness, angle perpendicular to the skin
Needle: 1 ½-inch, 22-gauge
Depth: 1 to 1 ½ inches
Volume: 3 to 4 mL anesthetic, 1 mL D80, or both
NOTE: Lightly advance the needle to feel the outer fascia, then enter the body of the muscle! Avoid triamcinolone because of the greater chance of atrophy of muscle or overlying subcutaneous tissue

Figure 1-1A Trigger point injection of the paracervical or upper trapezius muscles.

SUMMARY

Cervical strain is an irritation and spasm of the cervical and upper back muscles. Physical and emotional stress, dorsokyphotic posture, whiplash-like injuries, cervical arthritis, and underlying abnormal cervical alignment are common causes. Spinal nerve or spinal cord irritation or injury is a much less common cause of cervical strain.

TREATMENT OF CHOICE: Ice applications, a muscle relaxer at night for 7 to 10 days, and physical therapy exercises are the treatments of choice.

SEQUENCE OF TREATMENTS

1. Ice applied to the neck and upper back muscles reduces the acute muscular irritations.
2. *Exercise of choice:* Passive rotation stretching exercises are performed daily.
3. Neck massage is most effective after heating (manual, shower massager, etc.).
4. *Acute restrictions:* The head is maintained in neutral position, especially when sleeping; and rotation, bending, and flexion are minimized.
5. A muscle relaxer is prescribed for nighttime use only (a dosage enough to cause mild sedation).
6. *Most common immobilizer:* A soft Philadelphia collar is worn during the day for 2 weeks.
7. Gentle cervical traction is prescribed for resistant or chronic cases,
8. *Injection:* Local anesthetic with or without corticosteroid injection with depot methylprednisolone 80 mg/mL (D80) is used for severe, acute localized muscle irritation as seen with torticollis or whiplash or for refractory symptoms (see details on page 5).
9. *Recovery exercise:* Passive rotation stretching exercises with or without traction are performed after the acute symptoms have subsided.

SURGICAL PROCEDURE: None.

INJECTION: Local injection of anesthetic, corticosteroid, or both is used to treat the acute muscle spasm of torticollis and severe cervical strain, and to assist in the management of the acute flare-up of fibromyalgia. At best, its use is adjunctive to the physical therapy exercises.

Positioning: The patient is to be sitting up, with the shoulders back and the hands placed in the lap.

Surface Anatomy and Point of Entry: The midpoint of the superior trapezius is located halfway between the cervical spinous processes and the lateral aspect of the acromion. The paracervical muscles are located 1 inch lateral to the spinous processes.

Angle of Entry and Depth: The needle is inserted into the skin at a perpendicular angle. The depth is 1 to $1\frac{1}{2}$ inches.

Anesthesia: Ethyl chloride is sprayed on the skin. Local anesthetic is placed at the outer fascial plane (1 mL) and in the belly of the muscle (0.5 mL with each puncture).

Technique: The success of injection depends on the accurate placement of the most affected muscle. The point of maximum tenderness is palpated. The thick skin of the upper back is punctured rapidly. While holding the syringe as lightly as possible, the needle is passed through the subcutaneous layer until the tissue resistance of the outer fascia is met, approximately $\frac{3}{4}$ to 1 inch deep. (Note: The needle will not enter the muscle unless pressure is applied! Holding the syringe lightly will allow identification of the outer fascial layer.) One to 2 mL of local anesthetic is injected just outside the muscle. With firmer pressure, the needle is passed into the muscle belly, an additional $\frac{1}{4}$ to $\frac{3}{8}$ inch beyond the outer fascia. Often a "giving way" or "popping" will be felt as the fascia is penetrated; 1 to 2 mL of anesthetic, corticosteroid, or both is injected into an area the size of a quarter with three separate punctures. The second and third punctures are placed in a line that is perpendicular to the course of the muscle fibers. Restrict treatments to three injections per year to avoid "woody atrophy" of the muscle or the psychological dependence on injection!

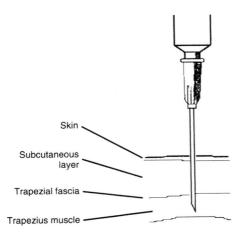

Skin

Subcutaneous layer

Trapezial fascia

Trapezius muscle

Figure 1-1B   Trapezius muscle injection.

INJECTION AFTERCARE
1. The injection site must be *protected for the first 3 days* by avoiding direct pressure, neck rotation, and lateral bending.
2. For severe cases, a soft Philadelphia *collar* should be used for 3 to 7 days.
3. *Ice* (15 minutes every 4 to 6 hours), *acetaminophen (Tylenol ES)* (1000 mg twice a day), or both, are used for postinjection soreness.
4. The upper back and neck are *protected for 30 days* by limiting neck rotation and lateral bending and by maintaining good posture.
5. Passive *rotation stretching exercises* are resumed at 2 to 3 weeks.
6. The injection can be repeated at 6 weeks if overall improvement is less than 50%.
7. If symptoms persist, *plain film radiographs* of the cervical spine are obtained to assess for the loss of normal cervical lordosis, the degree of underlying osteoarthritis, the presence of significant foraminal encroachment disease (reduction of 50% of the area of the foramina is significant), and for refractory cases.
8. An *MRI* is obtained to detect underlying cervical disk disease if patients fail to respond over the course of 2 to 3 months (less than 5% of cases are chronic).

OUTCOME AND FURTHER WORK-UP: Most episodes of cervical strain resolve completely with a combination of stress reduction, attention to posture, physical therapy, a short course of a muscle relaxer, and corticosteroid injection. However, because the muscle spasm of cervical strain represents a reaction to an underlying threat to the spinal column, cord, or nerve, any patient with recurrent or severe strain must be evaluated for underlying arthritis, disk disease, radiculopathy, spinal stenosis, and so forth. Patients suspected of reactive cervical strain should undergo plain film radiographs and MRI. Patients with diffuse muscular irritation of the cervical, thoracic, and lumbosacral spinal areas likely have fibromyalgia.

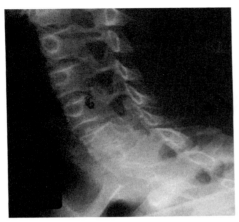

Large vertebral osteophytes narrowing the neuroforamina at the C6-C7 level—the seventh nerve

Figure 1-2 Cervical radiculopathy with vertebral osteophytes narrowing the exit foramina.

SUMMARY

Cervical radiculopathy is an impairment of the upper extremity neurologic function caused by compression of the spinal nerve, spinal cord, or both. Cervical arthritis with foraminal encroachment accounts for 90% of cases and a herniated nucleus pulposus accounts for nearly 10% of cases. Spinal stenosis, epidural abscess, epidural tumor, or primary spinal cord tumors are much less common causes. Severity is determined by the degree of functional impairment: sensory symptoms only (80% to 85%), sensorimotor symptoms with loss of spinal reflex, loss of motor strength, or muscle atrophy (15%), and spinal cord compression with long tract signs (less than 1%).

TREATMENT OF CHOICE: Ice applications, a muscle relaxer at night for 7 to 10 days, and physical therapy exercises are the treatments of choice.

SEQUENCE OF TREATMENTS

1. Ice is applied to the neck and upper back muscles for the acute muscular irritations.
2. *Exercise of choice:* Passive rotation stretching exercises are performed daily.
3. Neck massage is most effective after heating (manual, shower massager, etc.).
4. *Acute restrictions:* The head is maintained in neutral position, especially when sleeping; and rotation, bending, and flexion are minimized.
5. A muscle relaxer is prescribed for nighttime use only (a dosage enough to cause mild sedation).
6. *Most common immobilizer:* A soft Philadelphia collar is worn during the day for 2 weeks.
7. Gentle cervical traction is prescribed for resistant or chronic cases.
8. *Injection:* Local anesthetic with or without corticosteroid injection with D80 is used for severe, acute localized muscle irritation as seen with torticollis or whiplash or for refractory symptoms (see page 5).

9. **_Recovery exercise:_** Passive rotation stretching exercises with or without traction are performed after the acute symptoms have subsided.

SURGICAL PROCEDURE: Foraminotomy or diskectomy for persistent sensorimotor symptoms.

OUTCOME AND FURTHER WORK-UP: All patients with radiculopathy need plain films of the cervical spine to assess alignment, disk disease, and foraminal encroachment. Patients with advanced or progressive neurologic impairment (sensorimotor or sensorimotor with lower extremity long tract signs) must undergo MRI. The outcome of cervical radiculopathy depends on the degree of neurologic impairment, the length of time symptoms have been present, and the underlying diagnosis. The prognosis for sensory radiculopathy is uniformly good. Whether caused by foraminal encroachment or disk disease, a full recovery is expected. Sensorimotor radiculopathy, however, is a more extensive problem, is more likely to require surgical intervention, and is at greater risk for persistent symptoms from irreversible nerve damage.

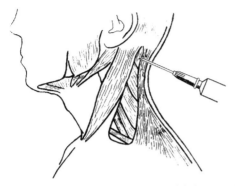

Enter 1 inch lateral to the midline and 1 inch caudal to the superior nuchal line of the skull (the base of the skull)
Needle: $1\frac{1}{2}$-inch, 22-gauge
Depth: $\frac{1}{2}$ to $\frac{3}{4}$ inch down to the fascia and then an additional $\frac{1}{4}$ inch into the muscle
Volume: 3 to 4 mL anesthetic, 1 mL D80, or both
NOTE: Lightly advance the needle to feel the outer fascia, then enter the body of the muscle! Avoid triamcinolone because of the increased tendency of muscle or subcutaneous atrophy

Figure 1-3A   Injection of the greater occipital nerve as it exits the semispinalis capitis muscle.

SUMMARY

Greater occipital neuritis is an isolated compression neuropathy of the greater occipital nerve as it courses from the upper cervical roots through the paracervical muscles to enter the subcutaneous tissue over the scalp. The nerve is composed solely of sensory fibers that provide pain, light touch, temperature, and vibration sensation to half of the scalp. Irritation and inflammation of the nerve occur as it penetrates the paracervical muscles. Patients complain of a unilateral headache, variable degrees of paresthesias or hypoesthesias, and symptoms reflecting cervical strain.

TREATMENT OF CHOICE: Treatment initiated with ice applications, a muscle relaxer prescribed at night for 7 to 10 days, and physical therapy stretching exercises of the cervical muscles are effective if begun promptly.

SEQUENCE OF TREATMENTS

1. Ice applied at the base of the skull effectively controls the acute muscular spasms.
2. *Exercise of choice:* Passive stretching exercises are performed daily.
3. Neck massage is most effective after heating (manual, shower massager, etc.).
4. *Acute restrictions:* Movement of the head is kept to a minimum, limiting rotation, bending, and flexion. In addition, the head is maintained in a neutral position with emphasis on keeping the head, neck, and torso aligned, especially at night while sleeping.
5. A muscle relaxer is prescribed for nighttime use only (a dosage enough to cause mild sedation).
6. *Most common immobilizer:* A soft Philadelphia collar helps to maintain good posture and assists in reducing the reactive muscle spasms.
7. *Injection:* Local anesthetic with or without corticosteroid injection with D80 is indicated for severe localized muscle irritation or refractory symptoms (see page 10).

SURGICAL PROCEDURE: None.

INJECTION: Local injection of anesthetic, corticosteroid, or both is used to treat the acute headache that has failed ice, a muscle relaxant or analgesic, and gentle stretching exercises.

Positioning: The patient is placed prone, with the head aligned with the torso.

Surface Anatomy and Point of Entry: The midline over the cervical spinous processes and the base of the skull are palpated and marked as appropriate (hairline!). The greater occipital nerve penetrates the paracervical muscles approximately 1 inch lateral to the spinous processes.

Angle of Entry and Depth: The needle is inserted into the skin at a perpendicular angle. The depth is $\frac{3}{4}$ to 1 inch down to the paracervical muscle fascia.

Anesthesia: Ethyl chloride is sprayed on the skin. Ask the patient to take several deep breaths before spraying the volatile liquid. Local anesthetic is placed at the outer fascial plane (1 mL) and just inside the belly of the muscle (1 mL).

Technique: The success of injection depends on the accurate placement of the anesthetic and corticosteroid above and below the fascial plane of the paracervical muscles. While holding the syringe as lightly as possible, the needle is passed through the subcutaneous layer until the moderate tissue resistance of the outer fascia is met, approximately $\frac{3}{4}$ to 1 inch in depth. (Note: The needle will not enter the muscle unless pressure is applied! Holding the syringe lightly will allow identification of the outer fascial layer.) Inject 1 to 2 mL of local anesthetic just outside the muscle. With firmer pressure, the needle is passed into the muscle belly, an additional $\frac{1}{4}$ to $\frac{3}{8}$ inch beyond the outer fascia. Often a "giving way" or "popping" will be felt as the fascia is penetrated. Alternatively, if the fascia is not readily identified as the needle is advanced, the proper depth can be confirmed by applying vertical traction to the overlying skin. If the needle is above the fascia, it should move freely in the dermis when applying skin traction! Similarly, the needle will stick in place if the tip has penetrated the fascia! Inject 0.5 to 1 mL of anesthetic, 0.5 mL of corticosteroid, or both above and below the fascia for optimal results.

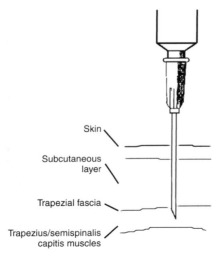

Skin

Subcutaneous
layer

Trapezial fascia

Trapezius/semispinalis
capitis muscles

Figure 1-3B   Greater occipital nerve injection.

10

INJECTION AFTERCARE

1. The injection site must be ***protected for the first 3 days*** by avoiding direct pressure, neck rotation, and lateral bending.
2. For severe cases, a soft Philadelphia ***collar*** should be used for 3 to 7 days.
3. ***Ice*** (15 minutes every 4 to 6 hours), ***acetaminophen*** (1000 mg twice a day), or both, are used for postinjection soreness.
4. The neck is ***protected for 30 days*** by limiting neck rotation, lateral bending, and maintaining good posture.
5. Passive ***rotation stretching exercises*** of the neck are resumed at 2 to 3 weeks.
6. The injection can be repeated at 6 weeks if overall improvement is less than 50%.
7. If symptoms persist, ***plain film radiographs*** or an ***MRI*** of the cervical spine are obtained to assess for the loss of normal cervical lordosis and the degree of underlying osteoarthritis or disk disease.
8. If the response to treatment is poor, a standard work-up for headaches should be undertaken.

OUTCOME AND FURTHER WORK-UP: Greater occipital neuritis is a self-limited condition. Anesthetic and corticosteroid injection is uniformly successful in the short term (relief lasting weeks or even a few months). However, long-term results demand attention to stress, posture, and physical therapy stretching exercises. Any patient who fails to respond to the sequence of treatments deserves a full work-up of the cervical spine and for chronic headaches.

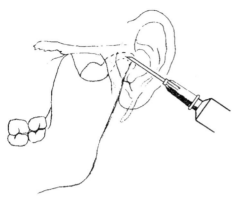

With the jaw fully opened, enter the joint $\frac{1}{4}$ to $\frac{3}{8}$ inch directly anterior to the tragus in the depression formed over the joint; angle perpendicular to the skin
Needle: $\frac{5}{8}$-inch, 25-gauge
Depth: $\frac{1}{4}$ to $\frac{1}{2}$ inch into the joint
Volume: 0.5 to 1 mL anesthetic, 0.5 mL K40, or both
NOTE: Identify the temporal artery by palpation, mark its course, and enter the skin on either side of it. Gently advance the needle into the joint. If arterial blood enters the syringe, exit the skin, hold pressure for 5 minutes, and reenter either slightly anterior or posterior to the artery

Figure 1-4A Injection of the temporomandibular joint.

SUMMARY

The temporomandibular joint (TMJ) is a hinge joint that is supported by two strong hinge ligaments (lateral temporomandibular ligament and the medial sphenomandibular ligaments), the muscles of mastication (medial and lateral pterygoid and the masseter muscles), and a thick joint capsule. In between the mandible and the temporal bone is a meniscal-like cartilage—the articular disk—located in the center of the joint. Arthritis of the joint is relatively uncommon. Post-traumatic osteoarthritis and rheumatoid arthritis are the most common causes of acute joint inflammation. TMJ syndrome is a recurring or chronic irritation of the joint secondary to malocclusion, nighttime grinding of teeth, and stress. Patients complain of pain when chewing, clicking, inability to open the mouth (pterygoid muscle spasm), or rarely a locked position of the jaw.

TREATMENT OF CHOICE: A liquid or mechanical soft diet is the treatment of choice for the acute symptoms arising from the joint. Stress reduction is the focus of attention when symptoms are subacute or chronic.

SEQUENCE OF TREATMENTS

1. A liquid or soft mechanical diet for 7 days is effective in relieving the acute pain and irritation.
2. Ice can be applied just anterior to the ear but is usually of limited benefit.
3. The nighttime use of a bite block protects the joint from the consequences of grinding of the teeth.
4. *Acute restriction:* Chewing meat, nuts, hard candy, and gum must be restricted to avoid aggravating the joint and the muscles of mastication.
5. A muscle relaxer taken at bedtime in a dosage enough to cause mild sedation should reduce the acute pterygoid and masseter muscle spasm and help curb the degree of grinding.
6. *Injection:* Local anesthetic, corticosteroid injection, or hyaluronic acid is indicated for refractory pain and impaired chewing.

12

7. **Recovery exercise:** The flexibility of the joint typically recovers gradually once the acute muscle spasm has been arrested. A minority of patients require passive stretching exercises.
8. **Consultation:** Referral to an oral surgeon who specializes in TMJ evaluation and treatment is suggested for patients with refractory symptoms.

SURGICAL PROCEDURE: None.

INJECTION: Local injection of anesthetic, corticosteroid, or hyaluronic acid is used to treat the acute arthritis.

Positioning: The patient is placed in the lateral decubitus position with a pillow supporting the head.

Surface Anatomy and Point of Entry: The tragus, temporal artery, and the articular tubercle of the zygomatic arch are palpated and marked. The patient is asked to open and close the mouth, feeling the concavity of the joint. The point of entry is directly over the center of the joint, halfway between the articular tubercle of the zygoma and the head of the mandible (the condylar process).

Angle of Entry and Depth: The needle is inserted into the skin perpendicularly. The depth is $\frac{3}{8}$ to $\frac{1}{2}$ inch.

Anesthesia: The patient is asked to take several deep breaths and then hold the breath. Ethyl chloride is sprayed on the skin. Local anesthetic is placed under the skin, just over the resistance of the joint capsule (0.5 mL), and intra-articularly (0.5 mL).

Technique: The success of injection depends on an intra-articular injection. The patient is asked to open the jaw to its maximum point. While holding the syringe as lightly as possible, the needle is slowly and carefully passed through the subcutaneous layer until the tissue resistance of the joint capsule is met, approximately $\frac{3}{8}$ to $\frac{1}{2}$ inch deep. If arterial blood enters the syringe, the needle is withdrawn, pressure is held for 5 minutes, and a point of entry either anterior or posterior to the

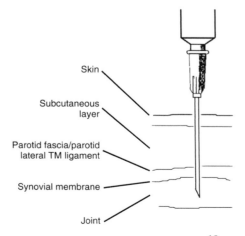

Skin

Subcutaneous layer

Parotid fascia/parotid lateral TM ligament

Synovial membrane

Joint

Figure 1-4B Temporomandibular (TM) joint injection.

13

artery is chosen. Inject 0.5 mL local anesthetic just outside the joint capsule. With firmer pressure, the needle is passed into the joint, an additional $\frac{1}{4}$ to $\frac{3}{8}$ inch beyond the joint capsule. Often a "giving way" or "popping" will be felt as the fascia is penetrated. Inject 0.5 mL of anesthetic, corticosteroid, or both intra-articularly. A successful injection reduces joint pain, allows freer opening and closing of the jaw, and decreases the acute pterygoid muscle spasm.

INJECTION AFTERCARE

1. The injection site must be *protected for the first 3 days* by avoiding direct pressure, chewing, and grinding of the teeth at night.
2. *Ice* (15 minutes every 4 to 6 hours), *acetaminophen* (1000 mg twice a day), or both, are used for postinjection soreness.
3. *Protect* the joint for 30 days by limiting chewing and grinding of the teeth at night.
4. A muscle relaxer taken at bedtime in a dosage enough to cause mild sedation should reduce the acute pterygoid and masseter muscle spasm and help curb the degree of grinding.
5. The injection can be repeated at 6 weeks if overall improvement is less than 50%.
6. Obtain *Panorex radiographs* of the teeth and mandible spine to assess for intrinsic pathology of the teeth, mandible and TMJ.
7. Obtain a *consultation* with an oral surgeon who specializes in TMJ disorders if treatment fails to provide long-term benefits.

OUTCOME AND FURTHER WORK-UP: More than 90% of patients with acute TMJ symptoms respond to a combination of restricted diet, jaw rest, and a muscle relaxer. Less than 10% of patients require injection. Patients with subacute or chronic TMJ symptoms should undergo special testing and consultation with an oral surgeon.

Chapter 2

SHOULDER

THE DIFFERENTIAL DIAGNOSIS OF SHOULDER PAIN

DIAGNOSES	CONFIRMATIONS
Rotator cuff syndromes (most common)	
Impingement syndrome	Passive painful arc
Rotator cuff tendinitis	Lidocaine injection test
Rotator cuff tendon thinning	Radiograph—shoulder series showing a narrow subacromial space
Rotator cuff tendon tear	Diagnostic arthrograms
Frozen shoulder	Loss of range of motion (ROM); normal shoulder radiograph, magnetic resonance imaging (MRI)
Acromioclavicular (AC) joint	
Osteoarthritis	Radiograph—shoulder series
AC separation	Radiograph—weighted views of the shoulder
Osteolysis of the clavicle	Radiograph—shoulder series
Subscapular bursitis	Local anesthetic block
Sternoclavicular joint	
Strain or inflammatory arthritis	Local anesthetic block
Septic arthritis (intravenous drug abuse)	Aspiration and culture
Glenohumeral joint	
Osteoarthritis	Radiograph—shoulder series (axillary view)
Inflammatory arthritis	Synovial fluid analysis
Septic arthritis	Synovial fluid culture
Multidirectional instability of the shoulder	
Dislocation	Radiograph—shoulder series
Subluxation	Abnormal sulcus sign
Glenoid labral tear	Double contrast arthrography
Referred pain	
Cervical spine	Neck rotation; radiograph; MRI
Lung	Chest radiograph
Diaphragm	Chest radiograph; computed tomography (CT) scan
Upper abdomen	Chemistries; ultrasound

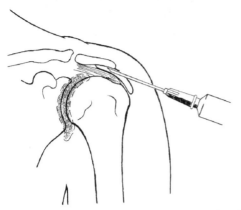

Enter 1 to 1½ inches below the
midpoint of the acromial process;
parallel the angle of the acromion to
the subacromial bursa
Needle: 1½-inch, 22-gauge
Depth: 1 to 1½ inches to 3½ inches
(obese patient)
Volume: 2 to 3 mL anesthetic and
1 mL D80
NOTE: Never inject under pressure or
if the patient experiences dramatic
pain (intratendinous or periosteal);
if pain develops or resistance to
injection is encountered, withdraw
½ inch and redirect (see page 17)

Figure 2-1 Subacromial bursal injection from the lateral approach.

SUMMARY

Impingement syndrome is the term used to describe the symptoms that result from the compression of the rotator cuff tendons and the subacromial bursa between the greater tubercle of the humeral head and the lateral edge of the acromion process. It is the "mechanical" component and principal cause of subacromial bursitis, rotator cuff tendinitis, rotator cuff tendon tear, and Milwaukee shoulder. Injection of the subacromial bursa provides rapid control of the inflammation caused by the pressure and friction of repeated impingement.

TREATMENT OF CHOICE: The weighted pendulum "stretch" exercise is performed daily to open the subacromial space and reduce the pressure on the rotator cuff tendons and subacromial bursa.

SEQUENCE OF TREATMENTS

1. Ice is applied anterolaterally over the deltoid muscle.
2. *Exercise of choice:* The weighted pendulum stretching exercise is performed twice a day.
3. *Acute restrictions:* Overhead positioning, overhead reaching, and lifting are restricted until the pain is substantially improved.
4. An oral nonsteroidal anti-inflammatory drug (NSAID) is prescribed in full dosage for 2 to 3 weeks.
5. *Injection:* A subacromial injection of anesthetic is used to determine the degree of accompanying tendinitis. If the patient's symptoms and signs are significantly improved with lidocaine, a corticosteroid is injected into the bursa (see page 17).
6. *Recovery exercise:* Isometrically performed external and internal rotation exercises are begun after the flexibility of the shoulder has improved significantly with the pendulum stretching exercise.
7. *Consultation:* Referral to a surgical orthopedist is appropriate for patients with refractory symptoms (3% to 5%).

SURGICAL PROCEDURE: Acromioplasty, performed arthroscopically or by open shoulder exposure, is the surgical procedure of choice for refractory impingement, especially in patients with severely down-sloping (type III acromions), greater tubercle bony erosions, or both.

INJECTION: Local injection of anesthetic or corticosteroid is used (1) to confirm the diagnosis of impingement or (2) to treat a subtle degree of rotator cuff tendinitis (see "Rotator Cuff Tendinitis," pages 18–20). If a subacromial bursal injection of anesthetic (the "lidocaine injection test") substantially reduces the patient's pain, improves the overall function of the shoulder, and significantly improves the abnormalities seen on examination (local tenderness and the painful arc maneuver), then corticosteroid injection can be performed.

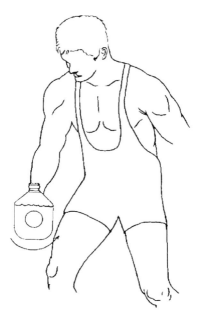

Figure 2-2   Weighted Pendulum Stretching Exercise—Regular use of this stretching exercise can increase the space under the acromion by $\frac{1}{4}$ inch, reducing the pressure on the subacromial bursa and rotator cuff tendons. It is the treatment of choice for the impingement syndrome and one of the primary treatments used in the treatment of rotator cuff tendinitis, bicipital tendinitis, frozen shoulder, osteoarthritis of the glenohumeral joint, and rotator cuff tendon tear. It is contraindicated in acromioclavicular separation, glenohumeral dislocation, and directional instability.

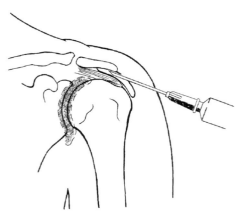

Enter 1 to 1½ inches below the midpoint of the acromial process; parallel the angle of the acromion to the subacromial bursa

Needle: 1½-inch, 22-gauge spinal needle

Depth: 1 to 1½ inches to 3½ inches (obese patient)

Volume: 2 to 3 mL anesthetic and 1 mL D80

NOTE: Never inject under pressure or if the patient experiences dramatic pain (intratendinous or periosteal); if pain develops or resistance to injection is encountered, withdraw ½ inch and redirect (see page 19)

Figure 2-3A   Subacromial bursal injection from the lateral approach.

SUMMARY

Rotator cuff tendinitis is an inflammation of the supraspinatus (abduction) and infraspinatus (external rotation) tendons lying between the humeral head and the acromial process. Repetitive overhead reaching, pushing, pulling, and lifting with the arms outstretched lead to compression ("subacromial impingement") and irritation of the tendons. The subacromial bursa, located just under the inferior surface of the acromion, functions to protect the tendons from the compressive forces of the two bones. Common shoulder tendinitis must be distinguished from frozen shoulder (loss of range of motion), rotator cuff tendon tear (persistent weakness), and biceps tendinitis (painful arm flexion).

TREATMENT OF CHOICE: The weighted pendulum stretching exercise combined with an effective anti-inflammatory treatment is the treatment of choice.

SEQUENCE OF TREATMENTS

1. Ice is applied anterolaterally over the deltoid muscle.
2. *Exercise of choice:* The weighted pendulum stretching exercise is performed twice a day.
3. *Acute restrictions:* Overhead positioning, overhead reaching, and lifting are restricted until the pain is substantially improved.
4. An oral NSAID is prescribed for 2 to 3 weeks.
5. *Injection:* The lidocaine injection test is used to differentiate the degree of mechanical impingement, active tendinitis, tendon tear (true weakness), or frozen shoulder (true stiffness). Once the patient's pain is controlled the actual degree of loss of strength or loss of range of motion can be more accurately determined! Injection of a long-acting corticosteroid is used to treat the active tendon inflammation or as an empiric treatment for chronic impingement (see page 19).

6. **Recovery exercise:** Isometrically performed external and internal rotation exercises are used to recover any lost rotation strength but must be delayed until substantial improvement in pain has occurred (typically at 2 to 3 weeks).
7. **Consultation:** Referral to a surgical orthopedist is suggested for patients with refractory symptoms (3% to 5%).

SURGICAL PROCEDURE: Acromioplasty for tendinitis with severe impingement.

INJECTION: Local injection of anesthetic and corticosteroid is used to (1) confirm the diagnosis of an uncomplicated rotator cuff tendinitis, (2) to treat active rotator cuff tendinitis that has persisted 6 to 8 weeks or that has failed to improve with steps 1 through 4 earlier, (3) to treat rotator cuff tendinitis that accompanies frozen shoulder, and (4) to palliate the symptoms of rotator cuff tendinitis that accompanies rotator cuff tendon tear in those patients unable to undergo a major surgical procedure.

Positioning: The patient is placed in the sitting position, with the hands placed in the lap. The patient is asked to relax the shoulder and neck muscles. If the patient is unable to relax, traction applied to the flexed elbow may be necessary to open the subacromial space.
Surface Anatomy and Point of Entry: The lateral edge of the acromion is located and its midpoint marked. The point of entry is 1 to $1\frac{1}{2}$ inches below the midpoint.
Angle of Entry and Depth: The angle of entry should **parallel** the patient's own acromial angle (averaging 50 to 65 degrees). The depth will vary according to the patient's weight and muscle development ($1\frac{1}{2}$ inches in an asthenic patient and up to $3\frac{1}{2}$ inches in an obese patient of more than 30% ideal body weight). Note that the depth and angle of injection can be measured directly off a posteroanterior shoulder radiograph with a metal marker placed at the point of entry!

Anesthesia: Ethyl chloride is sprayed on the skin. Local anesthetic is placed in the deltoid muscle (1 mL), the deep deltoid fascia (0.5 mL), and the subacromial bursa (1 to 2 mL). Note that the

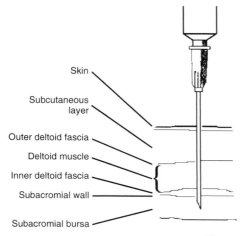

Skin
Subcutaneous layer
Outer deltoid fascia
Deltoid muscle
Inner deltoid fascia
Subacromial wall
Subacromial bursa

Figure 2-3B Subacromial bursal injection.

19

subacromial bursa will accept only 2 to 3 mL of total volume: If this volume is exceeded the medication will flow out of the bursa and down to the deltoid insertion at the mid humerus or along the superior border of the supraspinatus!

Technique: Successful treatment depends on the accurate injection of the subacromial bursa, using no greater than 3 mL of total volume. The **lateral approach** is most accessible and safest method. The intratendinous injection is nearly impossible when paralleling the angle of the acromion because the position of the needle is tangential to the tendon! The needle is advanced through the subcutaneous tissue and the deltoid muscle until the subtle resistance of the deep deltoid fascia is encountered. If firm or hard tissue resistance is encountered (deltoid tendon or periosteum, often painful), then the needle is withdrawn $\frac{1}{2}$ inch and the angle is redirected 5 to 10 degrees either up or down. A "giving way" or "popping" sensation is often felt when the subacromial bursa is entered. Following 1 to 2 mL of anesthesia, the patient's strength is tested again. If the patient's pain is significantly reduced and the strength of abduction and external rotation are within 75% to 80% of the unaffected side, then 1 mL of depot methylprednisolone 80 mg/mL (D80) is injected. *Never* inject under moderate to high pressure. If high injection pressure is encountered, first try rotating the syringe 180 degrees. If tension is still high and the patient is obviously anxious, ask the patient to take a deep breath and try to relax the shoulder muscles. If tension remains high, reposition the needle by $\frac{1}{4}$-inch increments or by altering the angle of entry by 5 to 10 degrees.

INJECTION AFTERCARE

1. The shoulder must be ***protected for the first 3 days***, avoiding direct pressure, reaching, overhead positioning, lifting, pushing, and pulling.
2. ***Ice*** (15 minutes every 4 to 6 hours), ***acetaminophen (Tylenol ES)*** (1000 mg twice a day), or both, are used for postinjection soreness.
3. The shoulder motion must be ***restricted for 30 days*** by limiting reaching, overhead positioning, lifting, pushing, and pulling.
4. Passively ***pendulum stretching exercise*** is resumed on day 4.
5. ***Isometric toning exercises*** of abduction and external rotation are begun at 3 to 4 weeks, after the acute pain and inflammation have resolved.
6. The ***injection*** can be repeated at 6 weeks if overall improvement is less than 50%.
7. ***Regular activities, work, and sports*** should be delayed until the lost muscle tone has been recovered by at least 75%.
8. Obtain plain film radiographs of the shoulder in all patients who experience less than 4 to 6 weeks of relief. Plain films of the shoulder are used to (1) measure the subacromial space distance (normal 10 to 11 mm), (2) assess the AC joint for inferior-directed osteophytes, or (3) identify signs of high-grade impingement (roughening or erosive changes at the greater tubercle). Obtain a shoulder MRI/arthrogram for patients at risk for rotator cuff tendon tear.

OUTCOME AND FURTHER WORK-UP: Corticosteroid injection must be combined with restriction of use, pendulum stretching exercise, and the recovery rotator toning exercises to maximize the outcome. Patients with persistent or progressive loss of flexibility require range of motion measurements and plain films of the shoulder to evaluate for frozen shoulder. Patients who fail to restore external rotation or abduction strength need plain films of the shoulder and MRI arthrography to evaluate for rotator cuff tendon tear.

RESULTS: Data collected in the Medical Orthopedic Clinic at Sunnyside Medical Center.

Table 2-1   Clinical Outcomes of Rotator Cuff Tendinitis after Subacromial Injection of Depo-Medrol 80 mg/mL (D80) (Diagnosis Confirmed with Local Anesthetic Block; 1 mL D80; Home Physical Therapy—Pendulum Stretching Exercises Plus Isometric Toning Exercises Performed Twice a Day; 18-Month Prospective Follow-up of 91% of Patients Enrolled)

	No. Patients (%)
Complete resolution	
One injection	48
Two injections 6 weeks apart	8
Total	56 (62%)
Recurrence (averaging 5-6 months after initial evaluation and treatment)	
Reinjected once	14
Reinjected twice	7
Multiple injections	3
Total	24 (27%)
Failed to respond; chronic tendinitis	7 (8%)
Rotator cuff tendon rupture (developed in the follow-up period)	3 (3%)*
Lost to follow-up	9
TOTAL	99

*Each of the cases of tendon rupture occurred after a significant injury. Two patients fell onto an outstretched arm (occurring at 6 weeks and 5 months) and one patient experienced a direct blow to the shoulder (occurring at 6 months). These three patients responded to further medical management. Surgical intervention was not required.

Table 2-2   Adverse Reactions to a Subacromial Injection of Depo-Medrol 80 mg/mL

	No. Patients (%)
None	48 (49%)
Pain	32 (33%)
Inflammatory flare reaction (pain, heat, swelling)	7 (7%)
Vasovagal reaction	4 (4%)
Bruise	4
Stiffness	2
Swelling, itching, nausea, flushing	1 each
Postinjection infection	0
Postinjection tendon rupture (within 6 weeks of injection)	1

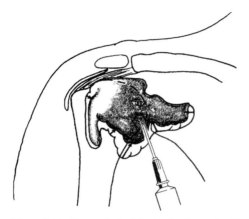

Frozen shoulder can be injected at the
subacromial bursa (see pages
19-20) or intra-articularly. The intra-
articular injection is inserted just
below the coracoid and is directed
outward (fluoroscopy is strongly
recommended when performing
dilation)
Needle: $1\frac{1}{2}$-inch or $3\frac{1}{2}$-inch spinal
needle, 22-gauge
Depth: $1\frac{1}{2}$ to $2\frac{1}{2}$ inches
Volume: 4 mL anesthetic, 10 to 12 mL
saline for dilation, and 1 mL K40

Figure 2-4A   Intra-articular injection for frozen shoulder.

SUMMARY

Frozen shoulder is a descriptive term that refers to a stiffened shoulder joint—a glenohumeral joint that has lost significant range of motion (abduction and rotation being most affected). Pathologically, the glenohumeral joint capsule has lost its normal distensibility. In long-standing cases, adhesions may form between the joint capsule and the humeral head (adhesive capsulitis). Rotator cuff tendinitis, acute subacromial bursitis, fractures about the humeral head and neck, and paralytic stroke are common causes.

TREATMENT OF CHOICE: Treatment always focuses on restoring the range of motion of the glenohumeral joint by passive stretching exercises. The weighted pendulum exercise is combined with passively performed glenohumeral stretching exercises with particular emphasis on the directions that have been affected most, typically external rotation and abduction.

SEQUENCE OF TREATMENTS

1. *Acute restrictions:* Active overhead positioning, overhead reaching, and lifting are restricted to avoid aggravating any underlying tendinitis or arthritis.
2. *Exercise of choice:* The weighted pendulum stretching exercise is combined with passive stretching exercises of the glenohumeral joint in external rotation and abduction and often are the only treatments necessary to resolve a mild to moderate case.
3. An oral NSAID is prescribed for 2 to 3 weeks (of limited benefit due to poor penetration).
4. *Subacromial injection:* A subacromial injection of D80 is indicated if inflammation of an underlying rotator cuff tendinitis persists or if the range of motion of the glenohumeral joint fails to improve over 6 to 8 weeks of physical therapy (see pages 19-20).
5. *Intra-articular injection:* Severe cases, those that have lost greater than 50% of external rotation, abduction, or both, are candidates for intra-articular injection of triamcinolone acetonide 40 mg/mL (K40) with or without concomitant glenohumeral joint saline dilation.

6. ***Recovery exercise:*** External and internal rotation isometric exercises are performed to recover the loss rotation strength and are begun when 75% of normal range of motion has been restored.
7. ***Consultation:*** Patients who fail to recover range of motion over 12 to 18 months—those who are refractory to stretching, subacromial and intra-articular injection, and saline dilation—are candidates for referral to a surgical orthopedist (1% to 2%).

SURGICAL PROCEDURE: Arthroscopic dilation of the glenohumeral joint and manipulation under general anesthesia are the most common procedures performed for refractory frozen shoulder (less than 2%).

INJECTION: A subacromial injection of corticosteroid is indicated when concurrent rotator cuff or bicipital tendinitis is present (see pages 19–20). A glenohumeral intra-articular injection combined with saline dilation is indicated when more than 50% of range of motion has been lost despite an adequate trial of physical therapy or subacromial injection.

Positioning: The patient should be recumbent with the head raised to 30 degrees.
Surface Anatomy and Point of Entry: The coracoid process is located and marked. The point of entry is $\frac{1}{2}$ to $\frac{3}{4}$ inch caudal to the coracoid.
Angle of Entry and Depth: The angle of entry is perpendicular to the skin and angled slightly outward. The depth is $1\frac{1}{2}$ to $2\frac{1}{2}$ inches. Fluoroscopy is strongly advised if dilation is performed.

Anesthesia: Ethyl chloride is sprayed on the skin. Local anesthetic is placed at the pectoralis major fascia (1 mL), the subscapularis fascia (1 mL), and the periosteum of the glenoid or humeral head (approximately 1 to 2 mL).
Technique: The successful treatment combines an intra-articular injection of corticosteroid with saline dilation of the joint. Fluoroscopy is recommended to ensure an accurate intra-articular injection. Ethyl chloride is sprayed on the skin. The needle is advanced to the firm resistance of

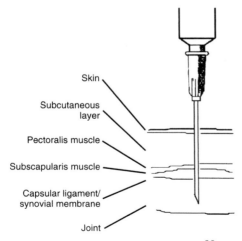

Skin
Subcutaneous layer
Pectoralis muscle
Subscapularis muscle
Capsular ligament/ synovial membrane
Joint

Figure 2-4B   Glenohumeral joint injection.

23

the pectoralis major fascia, the firm resistance of the subscapular fascia, and finally to the hard resistance of the periosteum of the shoulder. Anesthesia is placed at each tissue plane followed by 2 to 3 mL of radiopaque contrast to confirm the intra-articular position. Subsequently, 10 to 15 mL of normal saline is gradually injected. The volume will be determined by the increasing pressure to injection and the patient's awareness of a sense of tightening. At the completion of dilation, 1 mL of K40 is injected.

INJECTION AFTERCARE
1. The shoulder must be *protected for the first 3 days*, avoiding direct pressure, reaching, overhead positioning, lifting, pushing, and pulling.
2. *Ice* (15 minutes every 4 to 6 hours), *acetaminophen* (1000 mg twice a day), or both, are used for postinjection soreness.
3. The shoulder motion must be *restricted for 30 days* by limiting reaching, overhead positioning, lifting, pushing, and pulling.
4. The passively performed *weighted pendulum stretching exercise* as well as passively performed *stretching exercises* of abduction and external rotation are resumed on day 4.
5. *Isometric toning exercises* of abduction and external rotation are begun after 75% of normal range of motion has been restored.
6. An intra-articular *injection* can be repeated at 4 to 6 weeks if overall improvement is less than 50%.
7. *Regular activities, work, and sports* must be delayed until the majority of the shoulder's range of motion has been recovered and at least 75% of muscular tone has been restored.
8. *Consultation* with a surgical orthopedist is requested if the range of motion fails to increase by an average of 10% to 15% per month. Steady improvement in the range of motion can be assessed by the ability to rotate the shoulder and place the thumb on the spinous processes of the back. On average, the patient should be able to place the thumb 1 to 2 inches higher each month!

OUTCOME AND FURTHER WORK-UP: Frozen shoulder is a self-limiting condition. Given enough time and a rigorous daily physical therapy stretching program, shoulder flexibility will gradually return in the majority of patients. Most patients will recover 95% to 100% of their lost motion. However, patients with type 1 diabetes, those who have had difficulty performing physical therapy, and those with loss of range of motion approaching 50% of normal should be considered for glenohumeral joint dilation and corticosteroid injection. This procedure reduces pain, allows more active participation in physical therapy, and hastens the return to normal function.

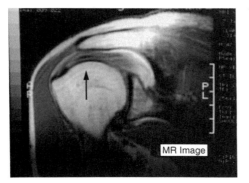

Transverse or longitudinal tendon tears occur at the musculoskeletal juncture—the anatomical area at risk for the greatest degree of impingement and the watershed area of poorest tendon blood flow

"Milwaukee shoulder": a combination of a large tendon tear, a large joint effusion, and radiographic changes of glenohumeral joint osteoarthritis

Diagnostic testing: plain film radiographs, shoulder arthrography, diagnostic ultrasound, or MRI

MR Image

Figure 2-5 Rotator cuff tendon tear (*arrow*, irregularity of the supraspinatus under the acromion).

SUMMARY

Rotator cuff tendon tears and loss of the normal integrity of the infraspinatus, the supraspinatus tendon, or both occur as the end result of chronic subacromial impingement, progressive tendon degeneration, acute traumatic injury, or a combination of these conditions. Risk factors for tendon disruption include (1) mucinoid degenerative tendon thinning, (2) injury from a fall or a direct blow to the shoulder, (3) age older than 62 years, (4) history of recurrent tendinitis, (5) a narrow "subacromial space" (normal width $\frac{1}{2}$ inch), and (6) weakness of external rotation, abduction, or both that is not attributable to the pain of active rotator cuff tendinitis, disuse atrophy, or suprascapular nerve irritation.

TREATMENT OF CHOICE: The treatment of choice varies according to age, the overall general health of the patient, and if the dominant side is affected! Surgical repair is recommended for the healthy 50- to 62-year-old worker with a large tear involving the dominant side. Long-term physical therapy, including passive stretching and active toning exercises is advised for the elderly patient with multiple medical problems (hence a poor surgical candidate) who has developed a "degenerative tear" occurring on the nondominant shoulder.

SEQUENCE OF TREATMENTS

Complete radiographic evaluation and surgical repair is strongly advised in the 50- to 65-year-old healthy patient with a moderate to large tear on the dominant side (greater than 50% loss of strength and inability to raise the arm over head without assistance). Medical treatment can be considered for the "partial" or small tears with modest loss of abduction and external rotation strength. Medical treatment includes the following:
1. Ice is applied over the anterolateral aspect of the deltoid muscle.
2. ***Immobilizer of choice:*** Continuous daytime use of the abduction pillow brace can be tried for 3 to 4 weeks.
3. ***Exercise of choice:*** The weighted pendulum stretching exercise is performed twice a day.
4. ***Acute restrictions:*** Overhead positioning, overhead reaching, lifting, pushing, and pulling are restricted until pain and strength have improved by at least 50%.

5. Isometric toning exercises in external rotation and abduction are performed carefully just to the edge of discomfort.
6. An oral NSAID can be prescribed at full dosage for 2 to 3 weeks but has limited benefit due to the mechanical nature of the problem.
7. *Injection:* The indications for local corticosteroid injection are very narrow given the fact that inflammation does not play a major role in this condition and corticosteroids may interfere with the healing process. Injection is mainly used to palliate the pain in the elderly patient who otherwise cannot or will not undergo surgical repair (see pages 19-20).
8. *Recovery exercise:* Isometrically performed external rotation and abduction exercises play a vital role in the recovery process whether treated surgically or medically.
9. For patients who fail to recover the loss of strength of rotation and abduction, long-term restrictions of reaching, pushing, pulling, and lifting are absolutely necessary.
10. *Consultation:* Patients with persistent functional impairment and refractory pain and swelling should be referred to a surgical orthopedist who specializes in shoulder repair and replacement.

SURGICAL PROCEDURE: Primary tendon repair with or without acromioplasty.

INJECTION: A subacromial injection of anesthetic is used to confirm the diagnosis of rotator cuff tendinitis complicated by tear (the lidocaine injection test demonstrating persistent weakness despite adequate control of pain!). Corticosteroid injection is used to reduce the pain and inflammation that can accompany the tear. In a limited number of patients, the control of the inflammatory component enables the patient to fully participate in the physical therapy recovery exercises. Corticosteroid injection can also be used to palliate the pain and swelling in the elderly patient who is unable to undergo surgical repair (see pages 19-20). In these cases, injection must be combined with immobilization to counter any adverse effect the corticosteroid may have on the healing process. An abduction pillow immobilizer or a simple shoulder immobilizer should be used concurrently for 30 days—the duration of action of the long-acting injectable corticosteroid.

OUTCOME AND FURTHER WORK-UP: As much as 15% of patients with rotator cuff tendinitis have tendon tears of various degrees (arthrographic data as well as the results of autopsy study). The vast majority of these tears heal as the active inflammation is relieved and the recovery exercises are completed. Less than 1% of these patients have profound weakness and dramatic loss of shoulder function suggesting large transverse tears. These patients require plain film radiographs and MRI to define the pathology and prepare for possible surgical repair.

RESULTS: These data were collected in the Medical Orthopedic Clinic at Sunnyside Medical Center.

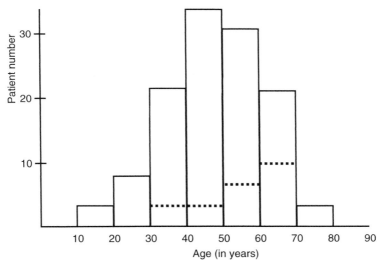

Figure 2-6 The results of Hypaque 60 subacromial bursography in 124 consecutive patients presenting with signs and symptoms of rotator cuff tendinitis. Of 124 cases, 104 patients were diagnosed as "uncomplicated" rotator cuff tendinitis (RCT) (average age, 57 years) and 20 had RCT complicated by tendon tears (average age, 67 years). N, 124; uncomplicated RCT, 104; RCT tears, 20 (dotted lines).

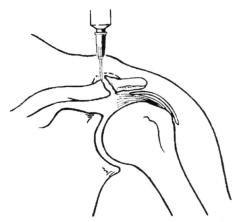

Enter just over the end of the clavicle (1$\frac{1}{2}$ inches medially to the lateral edge of the acromion)
Needle: $\frac{5}{8}$-inch, 25-gauge
Depth: $\frac{3}{8}$ to $\frac{5}{8}$ inch, down to the periosteum of the clavicle
Volume: 1 mL anesthetic and 0.5 mL K40
NOTE: The needle does not enter the joint directly! The injection is placed just under the synovial membrane attached to the distal clavicle

Figure 2-7A   Injection of the acromioclavicular joint at the distal clavicle just under the synovial membrane.

SUMMARY

The AC, coracoclavicular, and coracoacromial ligaments are attached tightly to the periosteum of their respective bones and hold the acromion, clavicle, and coracoid together. Falls to an outstretched arm, a dramatic blow to the anterior shoulder (tackling in football), or a fall landing directly on the anterior portion of the shoulder can cause the ligaments to be sprained, partially torn, or completely disrupted (first-, second-, and third-degree AC separations or sprains). Later in life, degenerative arthritis dominates the diagnoses at the AC joint. Over a lifetime of use, the articular cartilage wears down (normal width 3 to 5 mm), the bones become sclerotic, and bony osteophytes form on the ends of the clavicle and the acromion. Surprisingly, these nearly universal osteoarthritic changes cause symptoms in a very small percentage of the population (less than 5%).

TREATMENT OF CHOICE: Restriction of shoulder motion, including reaching, lifting, and avoiding direct pressure, is combined with applications of ice placed directly over the joint.

SEQUENCE OF TREATMENTS

1.   Ice is applied directly over the joint.
2.   *Acute restrictions:* Reaching overhead, adduction across the chest, and direct pressure (sleeping on the affected side) must be restricted until the pain and swelling have diminished by at least 50%.
3.   *Immobilizer of choice:* A Velcro shoulder immobilizer must be used for a minimum of 3 to 6 weeks for shoulder separation (less so for osteoarthritic flares).
4.   *Injection:* Local injection with anesthetic can be used confirm the diagnosis and differentiate it from bicipital or subscapularis tendinitis. Corticosteroid injection with K40 is used to treat osteoarthritis and first-degree sprains (see pages 29-30).

5. Recurrent or severe cases should be treated with the combination of corticosteroid injection and immobilization.
6. *Exercise of choice:* No single muscle supports the joint directly. General conditioning of the major shoulder muscles should minimize the stresses and strains of the joint.
7. Refractory cases may have to adhere to long-term restrictions of reaching, pushing, pulling, and lifting (military press, bench press, and pull-downs must be discontinued).
8. *Consultation:* Referral to a surgical orthopedist for persistent symptoms or severe functional impairment (impaired side sleeping, painful overhead reaching).

SURGICAL PROCEDURE: Second- and third-degree separations are most likely to remain symptomatic. A variety of stabilization procedures are available to eliminate the movement of the clavicle against the acromion. Distal clavicle resection remains the definitive procedure for arthritis (second- and third-degree separations) and for arthritis with inferiorly directed osteophytes that are encroaching on the rotator cuff tendons.

INJECTION: Local injection of anesthetic is used to confirm the diagnosis, in other words, to identify the AC joint as the source of the patient's symptoms rather than the rotator cuff tendons. Corticosteroid injection is used to control the symptoms of an acute arthritic flare or shoulder separation unresponsive to immobilization.

Positioning: The patient is placed in the sitting position with the shoulders held back and the hands in the lap.
Surface Anatomy and Point of Entry: The acromion and clavicle are identified. The AC joint is located either as a $\frac{1}{4}$-inch depression at the distal end of the clavicle or $1\frac{1}{2}$ inches medial to the lateral edge of the acromion. The point of entry is over the anterosuperior portion of the distal clavicle
Angle of Entry and Depth: A 25-gauge needle is inserted into the skin perpendicularly. The depth is $\frac{3}{8}$ to $\frac{5}{8}$ inch.

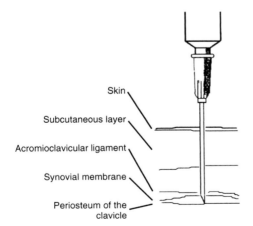

Skin

Subcutaneous layer

Acromioclavicular ligament

Synovial membrane

Periosteum of the clavicle

Figure 2-7B   Acromioclavicular joint injection.

Anesthesia: Ethyl chloride is sprayed on the skin. Local anesthetic is placed in the subcutaneous tissue (0.5 mL) and $\frac{1}{4}$ inch above the periosteum of the distal clavicle (0.5 mL). Note that the entire volume of anesthesia is injected $\frac{1}{4}$ inch above the joint, reserving the entire volume of corticosteroid for the joint!

Technique: This technique uses an **indirect method** of injecting cortisone into the joint, taking advantage of the anatomic attachment of the synovial membrane to the adjacent bone. The synovial membrane is approximately 1 cm long (see Fig. 2-7A). Instead of attempting to inject into the center of the joint, which is difficult, painful, and potentially dangerous (cartilage damage), a 25-gauge needle is advanced through the synovial membrane and down to the bone adjacent to the joint line. The center of the joint is *not* entered directly. After achieving anesthesia placed just above and outside the synovium, the needle is gently advanced down to the firm resistance of the periosteum of the clavicle. Using a separate syringe, the tip of the needle is held gently against the bone and 0.5 mL of K40 is injected. *Note:* The joint will not accommodate much medication. If the patient experiences increasing pressure, the needle should be withdrawn $\frac{1}{8}$ inch and the remaining steroid layered atop the joint, just outside the synovial membrane.

INJECTION AFTERCARE

1. The shoulder is ***protected for the first 3 days,*** avoiding overhead reaching, reaching across the chest, lifting, leaning on the elbows, and sleeping directly on it.
2. The use of a ***shoulder immobilizer*** is strongly encouraged to guard against displacement of the corticosteroid and to maximize the joint protection (optional).
3. ***Ice*** (15 minutes every 4 to 6 hours), ***acetaminophen*** (1000 mg twice a day), or both, are used for postinjection soreness.
4. The shoulder motion must be ***restricted for 30 days*** by limiting the movements listed in number 1 above.
5. Begin ***general shoulder conditioning*** at 3 to 4 weeks after the majority of pain and inflammation have resolved.
6. The ***injection*** can be repeated at 6 weeks if overall improvement is less than 50%; however, it is strongly advised to combine it with 3 to 4 weeks of immobilization.
7. ***Regular activities, work, and sports*** must be delayed until the pain has resolved and any lost strength from disuse has been restored.
8. ***Consultation*** with a surgical orthopedist is suggested if immobilization combined with two local injections is unsuccessful in resolving the condition.

OUTCOME AND FURTHER WORK-UP: The response to treatment depends on the degree of AC separation or extent of arthritis. Patients with first-degree AC separation or the early stage of arthritis respond well to injection and immobilization. Patients with second- and third-degree separations and advanced arthritic changes respond much less predictably. All patient should undergo plain films of both AC joints with and without weights to determine the stage of the problem.

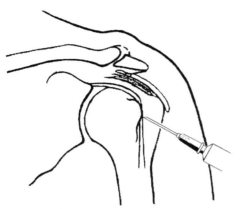

Enter 1 to 1¼ inches below the anterolateral corner of the acromion, directly over the bicipital groove

Needle: 1½-inch, 25-gauge

Depth: ½ to ¾ inch to either tubercle and ¾ to 1 inch to the bottom of the bicipital groove

Volume: 1 to 2 mL anesthetic and 1 mL D80

NOTE: Gently locate the periosteum of the tubercle, anesthetize the bone and carefully "walk down" the bone to the bottom of the groove.

CAUTION: Maintain the bevel of the needle parallel to the fibers of the tendon!

Figure 2-8A   Bicipital groove injection for bicipital tendinitis.

SUMMARY

Biceps tendinitis is an inflammation of the long head that results from the mechanical friction and irritation as the tendon moves back and forth in the bicipital groove of the anterior humerus. Repetitious lifting and to a lesser extent overhead reaching lead to a spectrum of pathologic changes that include simple inflammation, microtearing, chronic inflammation, mucinoid degenerative change, and tendon rupture. Risk factors for tendon rupture include (1) mucinoid degenerative change, (2) unusual or vigorous lifting injury, (3) age older than 62 years, and (4) a history of recurrent tendinitis.

TREATMENT OF CHOICE: Restriction of lifting is combined with ice applications placed over the anterior shoulder.

SEQUENCE OF TREATMENTS

1. Ice is applied over the anterior shoulder.
2. *Acute restrictions:* Upper extremity lifting of any degree and overhead reaching are restricted until the pain substantially subsides.
3. *Exercise of choice:* Because the long head tendon courses through the subacromial space to attach to the superior glenoid labrum, weighted pendulum stretching is the exercise of choice when tendon inflammation is still active.
4. An oral NSAID is prescribed in full dose for 2 to 3 weeks.
5. *Injection:* Local injection with anesthetic (to confirm the diagnosis), corticosteroid injection with D80 (to eliminate the acute inflammation), or both is indicated if the NSAID fails to control pain and inflammation.
6. *Recovery exercise:* Isometric strengthening of elbow flexion followed by active biceps curls is used to recover and enhance the strength of the short and long heads of the biceps as well as the brachioradialis muscles. These are begun after 50% of the pain and inflammation have subsided.

31

SURGICAL PROCEDURE: Surgery for bicipital tendinitis or bicipital tendon rupture is rarely indicated. Repair of the long head of the biceps is rarely necessary because the short head of the biceps and the brachioradialis provide 80% of the strength of flexion, and their combined strength can be enhanced by flexion exercises.

INJECTION: Several methods of injection can be used based on age and the risk of tendon rupture. Local injection of anesthetic placed directly into the bicipital groove is used to confirm the diagnosis of active tendinitis, and corticosteroid is used to treat the active inflammation. Because tendon rupture is rare in patients younger than age 50, bicipital groove injection—the most precise anatomic injection—is the preferred injection in this age group. However, with advancing age (older than 50 years) and especially in patients with recurring tendinitis, a subacromial bursal injection (see pages 19-20) or a glenohumeral intra-articular injection (see page 23) is preferred. These latter two injections avoid the hazard of direct needle penetration of the tendon associated with the bicipital groove injection.

Positioning: The patient is placed in the sitting position with the hands placed in the lap. The patient is asked to relax the shoulder and neck muscles.

Surface Anatomy and Point of Entry: The humeral head and the lateral edge of the acromion are located and marked. The point of entry is directly over the bicipital groove. It is located 1 to $1\frac{1}{4}$ inches caudal to the anterolateral edge of the acromion. When the examiner's fingers are over the anterolateral humeral head, the groove is palpable when the arm is passively rotated internally and externally.

Angle of Entry and Depth: The angle of entry is perpendicular to the skin. The depth is $\frac{1}{2}$ to $\frac{3}{4}$ inch to either bony prominence and $\frac{3}{4}$ to 1 inch to the bottom of the groove.

Anesthesia: Ethyl chloride is sprayed on the skin. Local anesthetic is placed at the firm tissue resistance of the lesser or greater tubercle (0.25 to 0.5 mL) and at the bottom of the bicipital groove (0.5 mL).

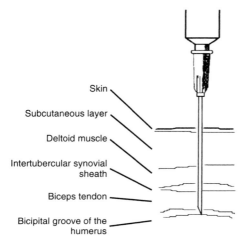

Skin

Subcutaneous layer

Deltoid muscle

Intertubercular synovial sheath

Biceps tendon

Bicipital groove of the humerus

Figure 2-8B   Bicipital tendinitis injection.

Technique: The success of treatment depends on the effective control of the inflammation of the bicipital tendon. If a **bicipital groove injection** is employed, it is imperative to maintain the bevel the needle parallel to the fibers of the tendon during the entire procedure! The needle is gently advanced down to the hard tissue resistance of the periosteum of either the lesser or greater tubercle, anesthetizing one or both. Having identified the adjacent bone, the needle is withdrawn $\frac{1}{4}$ to $\frac{3}{8}$ inch and redirected into the groove ($\frac{1}{4}$ inch deeper) until the "rubbery" firm resistance of the tendon or the hard resistance of the humerus is felt. Inject only under light pressure! Resistance when injecting suggests either an intratendinous or periosteal injection. If reexamination shows less local tenderness and less pain from isometric testing of arm flexion (greater than 50%), then 1 mL of D80 is injected.

INJECTION AFTERCARE

1. The upper extremity is ***protected for the first 3 days***, avoiding all lifting.
2. ***Ice*** (15 minutes every 4 to 6 hours), ***acetaminophen*** (1000 mg twice a day), or both, are used for postinjection soreness.
3. The tendon motion must be ***restricted for 30 days*** by avoiding, or at least limiting, lifting (held close to the body with low weight) and overhead reaching/positioning.
4. The passive weighted pendulum stretching exercise resumes on day 4.
5. Isometric elbow flexion exercises are begun after a substantial proportion of the pain has resolved.
6. The injection can be repeated at 6 weeks if overall improvement is less than 50% (accompanied by a discussion of the 10% chance of tendon rupture).
7. Regular activities, work, and sports must be delayed until the lost tone has fully been restored.

OUTCOME AND FURTHER WORK-UP: Bicipital tendinitis responds well to restricted use, the weighted pendulum stretching exercise, and corticosteroid injection. Ten percent of cases develop tendon rupture (the long head). Special radiographs or scans are not necessary to distinguish tendinitis from tendon rupture.

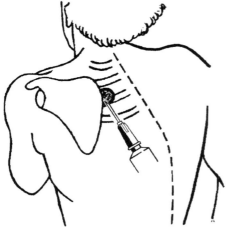

Enter directly over the second or third rib, whichever is closer to the superomedial angle of the scapula
Needle: $1\frac{1}{2}$-inch, 22-gauge
Depth: $\frac{3}{4}$ to $1\frac{1}{4}$ inches down to the periosteum of the rib
Volume: 1 to 2 mL anesthetic and 1 mL K40
NOTE: Place one finger above and one finger below the rib in the intercostal spaces and enter between these two; never advance more than $1\frac{1}{4}$ inches to avoid penetrating the parietal pleura of the lung

Figure 2-9A   Subscapular bursa injection.

SUMMARY

The subscapular bursa lubricates the underside of the scapula and the adjacent ribs. Inflammation of the bursa develops as a result of exaggerated movement of the scapula (mechanical pressure and friction develops between the superomedial angle of the scapula and the adjacent second and third ribs). Conditions that are associated with excessive scapular movement include frozen shoulder, glenohumeral osteoarthritis, and chronic rotator cuff tendinitis (with the gradual loss of normal glenohumeral movement, disproportionate degrees of shrugging occur). Mechanical pressure and friction can also occur in thin patients with poor muscular development, patients with dorsokyphotic posture, workers that perform repetitive to-and-fro motion of the upper extremities (ironing, assembly work, etc.), and athletes who perform heavy bench press exercises.

TREATMENT OF CHOICE: Corticosteroid injection with K40.

SEQUENCE OF TREATMENTS
1. Maintaining upright posture is emphasized.
2. *Acute restrictions:* Reaching across the chest and direct pressure against the back such as in reclining against hard surfaces must be avoided.
3. *Exercise of choice:* Isometrically performed internal rotation and adduction toning exercises to enhance the tone and bulk of the subscapularis muscle should be performed daily.
4. *Injection:* Local injection of anesthetic to distinguish subscapular bursitis from rhomboid or trapezial muscle irritation is always indicated when the two coexist, and injection with corticosteroid with K40 when pain and inflammation have been present for several weeks.
5. *Recovery exercises:* Isometric toning of internal rotation and adduction to enhance the tone and bulk of the subscapularis muscle may prevent future episodes of bursitis.

SURGICAL PROCEDURE: None.

INJECTION: Local injection of anesthetic is used to confirm the diagnosis, and a corticosteroid is used to treat the active inflammation. NSAIDs are not effective for this condition because of poor tissue penetration.

Positioning: The patient is placed in the sitting position. In order to fully expose the bursa, the shoulder on the affected side is fully adducted and the patient is asked to place the hand on the contralateral shoulder.

Surface Anatomy and Point of Entry: The superomedial angle of the scapula is identified. With the shoulder fully adducted, the second and third ribs are identified and marked. With one finger in the intercostal space above and one finger in the intercostal space below, the needle is inserted directly over the rib.

Angle of Entry and Depth: The angle of entry is perpendicular to the skin. The depth is $\frac{3}{4}$ inch in thin patients and up to $1\frac{1}{4}$ inches in heavier patients. Caution: *Never* advance deeper than $1\frac{1}{4}$ inches to avoid puncturing the parietal pleura of the lung! If periosteum has not been encountered at $1\frac{1}{4}$ inches, withdraw the needle and redirect!

Anesthesia: Ethyl chloride is sprayed on the skin. Local anesthetic is placed at the firm tissue resistance of the periosteum of the rib (1 to 2 mL). Minimize the amount of anesthesia placed in the muscular layer above the rib so as to distinguish the pain arising from the bursa from any associated involvement of the overlying levator scapulae and rhomboid muscles.

Technique: The successful injection of the bursa depends on the proper positioning of the patient and the accurate placement of medication at the level of the periosteum of the rib. The needle is advanced through the trapezius and the rhomboid muscles to the hard resistance of the periosteum of the rib. Alternatively, the needle is advanced no greater than $\frac{3}{4}$ inch beyond the outer fascia of the trapezius if the hard resistance of the periosteum of the rib cannot be positively identified (the trapezius and the rhomboid muscles are approximately $\frac{3}{8}$ inch thick each, total $\frac{3}{4}$ inch). Both the anesthetic and the corticosteroid are injected at the level of the periosteum.

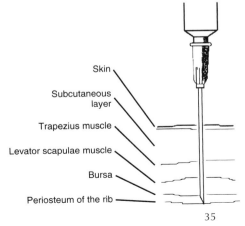

Skin

Subcutaneous layer

Trapezius muscle

Levator scapulae muscle

Bursa

Periosteum of the rib

Figure 2-9B Subscapular bursa injection.

INJECTION AFTERCARE

1. All direct pressure over the upper back and to-and-fro shoulder motions must be *avoided for the first 3 days*.
2. *Ice* (15 minutes every 4 to 6 hours), *acetaminophen* (1000 mg twice a day), or both, are used for postinjection soreness.
3. The upper back and shoulder motion must be *restricted for 30 days* by limiting direct pressure and the extremes of shoulder motion.
4. Upright *posture* must be maintained.
5. *Isometric toning exercises* of internal rotation and adduction are begun at 3 weeks (if the bulk and tone of the subscapularis muscle can be increased, the scapula will be less likely to rub against the underlying ribs).
6. The *injection* can be repeated at 6 weeks if overall improvement is less than 50%.
7. *Regular activities, work, and sports* must be delayed until the pain and inflammation have resolved and improvement in adduction and internal rotation strength has increased substantially.

OUTCOME AND FURTHER WORK-UP: Subscapular bursitis responds dramatically to a properly placed corticosteroid at the level of the adjacent rib. In order to avoid recurrences and to ensure a long-term benefit, a full exam of the glenohumeral joint and neck is performed to identify any underlying cause. Shoulder and cervical plain films are used to identify underlying glenohumeral joint arthritis, chronic rotator cuff tendinitis with thinning, degenerative cervical disk disease, and so forth.

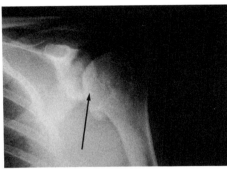

Intra-articular injection enters $\frac{1}{2}$ inch below the coracoid process and is directed outward and upward toward the medial portion of the humeral head (see page 23)
Needle: $1\frac{1}{2}$-inch or $3\frac{1}{2}$-inch spinal needle, 22-gauge
Depth: $1\frac{1}{2}$ to $2\frac{1}{2}$ inches, down to periosteum of the humeral head or glenoid
Volume: 3 to 4 mL anesthetic and 1 mL K40
NOTE: Fluoroscopy is strongly recommended in obese patients

Figure 2-10   Intra-articular injection of the shoulder (*arrow*, direction of injection).

SUMMARY

Osteoarthritis of the glenohumeral joint—a wear-and-tear of the articular cartilage of the glenoid labrum and humeral head—is an uncommon problem. In most cases, trauma precedes the condition, although the injury may have occurred years or decades earlier. Injuries that are associated with the development of osteoarthritis include previous dislocation, humeral head or neck fracture, large rotator cuff tendon tears (loss of musculotendinous support), and rheumatoid arthritis. Plain film radiographs demonstrate osteophyte formation on the inferior portion of the humeral head, flattening and sclerosis of the humeral head, and narrowing of the inferior portion of the glenohumeral articular cartilage (normal 3 to 4 mm).

TREATMENT OF CHOICE: Physical therapy exercises are the first line treatments and include the weighted pendulum stretching exercise and isometric toning exercises of external rotation and abduction combined with restricted use.

SEQUENCE OF TREATMENTS

1. Ice is applied over the anterior joint.
2. *Acute restrictions:* Reaching in any direction and lifting are restricted.
3. *Exercise of choice:* The weighted pendulum stretching exercise performed daily will reduce the pressure between the humeral head and the glenoid.
4. An NSAID in full dose is prescribed for 3 to 4 weeks.
5. *Most common immobilizer:* A Velcro shoulder immobilizer can be used with caution for severe arthritic flare (daily stretching exercises must accompany the use of immobilization to guard against the development of frozen shoulder).
6. *Injection:* Local corticosteroid injection with K40 is used if the NSAID fails to control pain and inflammation (see details, page 23).
7. *Recovery exercise:* Isometrically performed external and internal rotation toning exercises to provide support to the joint are performed when pain and inflammation are controlled.
8. *Consultation:* Consultation with an orthopedic surgeon specializing in shoulder replacement is appropriate when pain is uncontrolled and significant shoulder function has been lost.

SURGICAL PROCEDURE: Shoulder replacement (arthroplasty) is indicated when pain is intractable and when 50% of the normal range of motion of the shoulder has been lost.

INJECTION: Local injection of anesthetic is used to confirm the diagnosis (to separate it from concurrent rotator cuff disease, for example). Corticosteroid injection is used to control the symptoms of the acute arthritic flare (see page 23).

OUTCOME AND FURTHER WORK-UP: Intra-articular injection and oral steroids provide temporary benefit at best for glenohumeral arthritis. Radiographs are necessary to determine the severity of the problem. Surgery remains the treatment of choice.

The treatment of choice is isometric toning exercises of internal and external rotation with the shoulder kept in neutral position; resistance is accomplished using a Thera-Band, bungee cord, an inner tube, and the like.

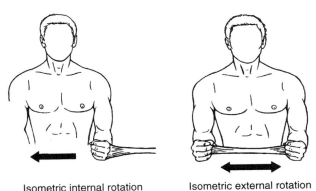

Isometric internal rotation   Isometric external rotation

Figure 2-11   Multidirectional instability of the shoulder.

SUMMARY

Multidirectional instability of the shoulder is synonymous with "subluxation," "loose" shoulder, or partial dislocation. It is more common in young women with poor muscular development, patients with large rotator cuff tendon tears (loss of muscular support), and athletic patients younger than the age of 40, especially swimmers and throwers. The examination of the shoulder includes the following abnormal signs: (1) the "sulcus sign" when downward traction is applied to the upper arm, (2) translocation of the humeral head in the glenoid fossa when applying force in the anteroposterior direction, (3) variable degrees of crepitation or popping, and (4) apprehension when performing the extremes of range of motion (especially rotation). This abnormal movement places the shoulder at risk for rotator cuff tendinitis. Nonsurgical treatment involves (1) maximizing the tone and strength of the infraspinatus and subscapular tendons (internal and external rotation isometric toning exercises) to enhance the support to the glenohumeral joint, (2) restricting reaching and lifting, and (3) treating any concurrent rotator cuff tendinitis.

TREATMENT OF CHOICE: Isometrically performed internal and external rotation toning exercises are combined with restricted reaching and lifting.

SURGICAL PROCEDURE: Several variations of the Putti Platt procedure involve the removal of redundant capsule and reinforcement of the anterior joint capsule utilizing the subscapularis tendon. Each of the procedures strives to achieve greater stability of the joint while attempting to avoid excessive tightening of the joint (loss of range of motion or impaired muscle strength).

INJECTION: Corticosteroid injection is indicated if instability is complicated by rotator cuff or bicipital tendinitis (see pages 19-20).

OUTCOME AND FURTHER WORK-UP: Physical therapy strengthening exercises in internal and external rotation are the principal means of reducing the frequency of dislocation and degree of subluxation. Unless the patient has a complicating rotator cuff tendinitis, NSAIDs and corticosteroid injection are not indicated. Patients experiencing anterior shoulder pain, limited range of motion, and clicking arising from the glenohumeral joint should undergo shoulder radiographs and MRI. Radiographic studies are necessary to fully define secondary glenoid labral tears, anterior glenoid rim fractures, rotator cuff tendon tears, and the degree of glenohumeral osteoarthritis.

Chapter 3

ELBOW

THE DIFFERENTIAL DIAGNOSIS OF ELBOW PAIN

DIAGNOSES	CONFIRMATIONS
Lateral epicondylitis (most common)	Local anesthetic block
Brachioradialis muscle strain	Examination
Medial epicondylitis	Local anesthetic block
Olecranon bursitis	
Draftsman's elbow	Aspiration; hematocrit
Septic bursitis	Aspiration; Gram stain/culture
Bursitis secondary to gout	Aspiration; crystal analysis
Hemorrhage secondary to chronic renal failure	Aspiration; hematocrit; chemistries
Olecranon spur fracture	Radiographs: elbow series
Triceps tendinitis	Examination
Radiohumeral arthritis	
Osteochondritis dissecans	Radiographs; magnetic resonance imaging (MRI); surgical exploration
Post-traumatic osteoarthritis	Radiographs: elbow series
Inflammatory arthritis	Aspiration; cell count
Hemarthrosis	Aspiration; hematocrit
Cubital tunnel	Nerve conduction velocity testing
Bicipital tendinitis	Local anesthetic block
Referred pain	
Cervical spine	Neck rotation; radiograph; MRI
Carpal tunnel syndrome	Nerve conduction velocity testing
Shoulder tendinitis	Painful arc; subacromial tenderness; isometric testing of the tendons

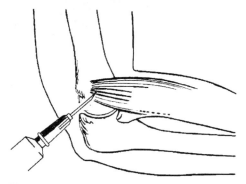

Enter directly over the prominence of the lateral epicondyle; use skin traction to identify the interface of the subcutaneous fat and the extensor carpi radialis tendon!
Needle: $^5/_8$-inch, 25-gauge
Depth: $^1/_4$ to $^1/_2$ inch, just above the tendon
Volume: 1 to 2 mL anesthetic and 0.5 mL D80
NOTE: *Never* inject under forced pressure or if the patient experiences sharp pain (too deep and likely intratendinous!)

Figure 3-1A Injection for lateral epicondylitis at the interface of the dermis and tendon.

SUMMARY

Lateral epicondylitis (tennis elbow) is an injury of the common extensor tendons (most commonly extensor carpi radialis brevis) at the origin at the lateral epicondyle of the humerus. Unaccustomed or repetitive lifting, tooling, hammering, or sports activities involving tight gripping and repetitive impact cause microtearing, microsplitting, or microavulsion of the tendon(s). Secondary inflammation develops at the epicondyle after this mechanical injury.

TREATMENT OF CHOICE: Ice placed over the lateral epicondyle is combined with immobilization of the wrist to prevent traction and tension at the elbow!

SEQUENCE OF TREATMENTS

1. *Most common immobilizer:* Mild to moderate symptoms respond to a Velcro wrist immobilizer with metal stay.
2. Ice is as effective as the nonsteroidal anti-inflammatory drug (NSAID) treatment applied directly to the lateral epicondyle.
3. *Acute restrictions:* Lifting, tooling, hammering, and forearm supination and pronation must be avoided to reduce the tension and traction across the tendons.
4. An oral NSAID in full dosage for 2 to 3 weeks has limited benefit because of poor tissue penetration.
5. *Immobilizer for severe tendinitis:* A short arm cast or long arm posterior splint is recommended for patients with severe symptoms to protect the tendon against any tension or traction.
6. *Injection:* Local corticosteroid injection with depot methylprednisolone 80 mg/mL (D80) is combined with continued immobilization (see page 43).
7. Long arm casting is used for severe cases, those with a loss of more than half of grip strength.
8. *Recovery exercises:* Isometrically performed gripping exercises followed by wrist extension exercises are begun after the acute signs and symptoms have significantly improved.
9. *Regular activities, work, and sports* must be delayed until the forearm muscular tone and strength have been restored.
10. The tennis elbow band is used for prevention.

SURGICAL PROCEDURE: Tendon excision, débridement, tendon lengthening, and tenotomy are procedures used for refractory cases. Those patients failing to improve with two courses of immobilization combined with injection can be considered for surgical repair.

INJECTION: Local injection with a corticosteroid is indicated when initial management with immobilization fails to reduce symptoms sufficiently to allow participation in the physical therapy recovery exercises.

Positioning: The patient is placed in the supine position, the elbow is flexed to 90 degrees, and the hand is placed under the ipsilateral buttock (for maximum exposure of the epicondyle).

Surface Anatomy and Point of Entry: The lateral epicondyle is most prominent and readily palpated with the elbow flexed to 90 degrees. It is located $\frac{1}{2}$ inch proximal to the radial head (the radial head should rotate smoothly under the examiner's fingers when passively supinating and pronating the forearm). The point of entry is directly over the center of the epicondyle.

Angle of Entry and Depth: Most patients have little subcutaneous tissue overlying the epicondyle. The depth down to the interface of the dermis and the extensor tendons averages $\frac{1}{4}$ to $\frac{3}{8}$ inch but can be as superficial as $\frac{1}{8}$ inch. With so little overlying subcutaneous fat, it is necessary to create a space for the corticosteroid injection by pinching up the skin, entering the tented-up skin at an angle, and distending the area with 1 mL of anesthetic.

Anesthesia: Ethyl chloride is sprayed on the skin. Local anesthetic is placed in the subcutaneous tissue only (0.5 mL).

Technique: The successful injection requires the accurate placement of the medication at the interface of the subcutaneous fat and the tendon. The depth of injection can be accurately determined either by gradually advancing the needle until the patient feels mild discomfort (the subcutaneous tissue is usually pain free) or until the rubbery tissue resistance of the tendon is felt.

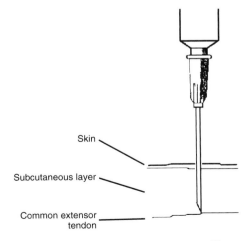

Skin

Subcutaneous layer

Common extensor tendon

Figure 3-1B Lateral epicondylitis injection.

43

Note: A painful reaction to injection or firm resistance during injecting suggests the needle is too deep and within the body of the tendon. Alternatively, the proper depth can be confirmed by applying vertical traction to the overlying skin. If the needle is properly placed above the tendon, it should move freely in the dermis when applying skin traction! Similarly, the needle will stick in place if the tip has penetrated the body of the tendon! In the latter case, simply withdraw the needle $\frac{1}{8}$ inch. The corticosteroid should always be injected at the interface between the subcutaneous fat and the tendon!

INJECTION AFTERCARE

1. The elbow must be ***protected for the first 3 days*** by avoiding all lifting, typing, writing, turning of the forearms, hammering, and direct pressure over the epicondyle.
2. ***Ice*** (15 minutes every 4 to 6 hours), ***acetaminophen (Tylenol ES)*** (1000 mg twice a day), or both, are used for postinjection soreness.
3. The elbow motion must be ***restricted for 3 to 4 weeks*** by the uninterrupted use of the Velcro wrist brace or a short arm cast and by avoiding direct pressure over the epicondyle. Because neither device sufficiently restricts forearm supination or pronation, the examiner must emphasize restricting of turning of door handles, keys, and so forth.
4. Begin ***gripping exercises*** at half tension after the immobilization phase. Begin with a half grip—just enough to firm the forearm muscles—and gradually build up over 1 to 2 weeks.
5. With restoration of normal grip strength, ***isometric toning exercises of wrist extension*** are begun at low tension and slowly increased. The patient should exercise only to the edge of discomfort; patients experiencing forearm muscle soreness are probably exercising too aggressively. Exercises must be interrupted if the lateral epicondyle becomes progressively more irritated.
6. The ***injection*** can be repeated at 6 weeks if improvement in pain, tenderness, or strength is less than 50% and especially if the recovery exercises listed here are poorly tolerated.
7. ***Regular activities, work, and sports*** must be delayed until the pain and inflammation have resolved and grip and wrist extension strength have increased substantially.
8. Long-term recommendations emphasize the need to perform "*palms-up*" lifting, a wrist bar when typing, thick, padded grips for tools, and any other changes that would lessen the direct traction or direct pressure on the outer elbow tendons.
9. Obtain ***plain film radiographs*** of the elbow and consider a ***consultation with a surgical orthopedist*** for patients with chronic symptoms.

OUTCOME AND FURTHER WORK-UP: Ninety-five percent of patients respond to a combination of rest and restricted use, wrist immobilization, and corticosteroid injection. The remaining 5% may respond to long-term physical therapy toning exercises with severe restrictions of forearm use. Patients failing to restore forearm and wrist function (chronic tendinitis—mucinoid degeneration of the tendon) can be considered for surgical exploration and tendon repair.

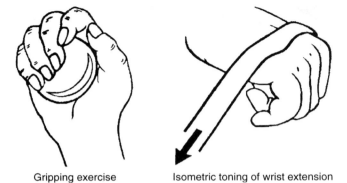

Gripping exercise   Isometric toning of wrist extension

Figure 3-2   Isometric Toning Exercises of the Forearm Muscles—After an effective anti-inflammatory response at the epicondyle and 3 weeks of rest and protection (wrist brace, short arm cast, etc.), isometric toning of the flexors and extensors of the forearm is performed to complete the treatment of epicondylitis.

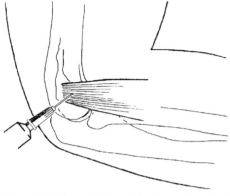

Enter $^3/_8$ to $^1/_2$ inch distal to the prominence of the medial epicondyle; use skin traction to identify the interface between the subcutaneous fat and the tendon!

Needle: $^5/_8$-inch, 25-gauge

Depth: $^1/_4$ to $^1/_2$ inch, just above the tendon

Volume: 1 to 2 mL anesthetic and 0.5 mL D80

NOTE: *Never* inject under forced pressure or if the patient experiences sharp pain (too deep within the tendon)

Figure 3-3A Injection for medial epicondylitis at the interface of the dermis and the tendon.

SUMMARY

Medial epicondylitis (golfer's elbow) is an injury of the common flexor tendons (most commonly flexor carpi radialis brevis) at the medial epicondyle of the humerus. Unaccustomed or repetitive lifting, tooling, hammering, or sports activities involving gripping and impact cause microtearing, microsplitting, or microavulsion of the tendon(s). Secondary inflammation develops at the epicondyle after this mechanical injury.

TREATMENT OF CHOICE: Ice placed over the medial epicondyle is combined with immobilization of the wrist to prevent traction and tension at the elbow.

SEQUENCE OF TREATMENTS

1. *Most common immobilizer:* A Velcro wrist brace with metal stay is effective for mild to moderate tendinitis (it reduces 75% to 80% of the forearm tension generated by the wrist).
2. Ice is applied directly to the medial epicondyle.
3. *Acute restrictions:* Lifting, tooling, hammering, and forearm supination and pronation must be avoided to reduce the tension and traction across the tendons!
4. An oral NSAID in full dosage for 2 to 3 weeks has limited benefit because of poor tissue penetration.
5. *Immobilizer for severe tendinitis:* A short arm cast or long arm posterior splint is recommended for patients with severe symptoms to protect the tendon against any tension or traction.
6. *Injection:* Local corticosteroid injection with D80 is combined with continued immobilization (see details on page 47).
7. Long arm casting is used for the most resistant cases.
8. *Recovery exercises:* Isometrically performed gripping exercises followed by wrist extension exercises are begun after the acute signs and symptoms have been significantly improved.

9. ***Regular activities, work, and sports*** must be delayed until the forearm muscular tone and strength have been restored.
10. The tennis elbow band is used for prevention.

SURGICAL PROCEDURE: Tendon débridement or tendon lengthening can be considered in patients that fail to improve with two courses of immobilization and injection.

INJECTION: Local injection with a corticosteroid is indicated when the initial management with immobilization fails to reduce symptoms sufficiently to allow participation in the physical therapy recovery exercises.

Positioning: The patient is placed in the supine position, the elbow is flexed to 90 degrees, and the arm is rotated externally as far as comfortable.

Surface Anatomy and Point of Entry: The medial epicondyle is most prominent and readily palpated with the elbow flexed to 90 degrees. The point of entry is $\frac{1}{2}$ inch distal to the center of the epicondyle.

Angle of Entry and Depth: Most patients have little subcutaneous tissue overlying the epicondyle. The depth down to the interface of the dermis and the extensor tendons averages $\frac{1}{4}$ to $\frac{3}{8}$ inch but can be as superficial as $\frac{1}{8}$ inch. With so little overlying subcutaneous fat, it is necessary to create a space for the corticosteroid injection by pinching up the skin, entering the tented-up skin at an angle, and distending the area with 1 mL of anesthetic.

Anesthesia: Ethyl chloride is sprayed on the skin. Local anesthetic is placed in the subcutaneous tissue only (0.5 mL or up to 1 mL) to create a greater space for the steroid.

Technique: The successful injection requires the accurate placement of the medication at the interface of the subcutaneous fat and the tendon. The depth of injection can be accurately determined either by gradually advancing the needle until the patient feels mild discomfort (the

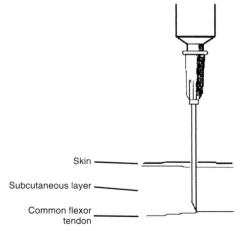

Skin

Subcutaneous layer

Common flexor tendon

Figure 3-3B   Medial epicondylitis injection.

subcutaneous tissue is usually pain free) or until the rubbery tissue resistance of the tendon is felt. Note that a painful reaction to injection or firm resistance during injecting suggests the needle is too deep and within the body of the tendon. Alternatively, the proper depth can be confirmed by applying vertical traction to the overlying skin. If the needle is properly placed above the tendon, it should move freely in the dermis when applying skin traction! Similarly, the needle will stick in place if the tip has penetrated the body of the tendon! In the latter case, simply withdraw the needle $\frac{1}{8}$ inch. The corticosteroid should always be injected at the interface between the subcutaneous fat and the tendon!

INJECTION AFTERCARE
1. The elbow must be *protected for the first 3 days* by avoiding all lifting, typing, turning of the forearms, tooling, hammering, and direct pressure.
2. *Ice* (15 minutes every 4 to 6 hours), *acetaminophen* (1000 mg twice a day), or both, are used for postinjection soreness.
3. The elbow must be *protected for 3 to 4 weeks* by the uninterrupted use of the Velcro wrist brace or a short arm cast and by avoiding direct pressure over the epicondyle. Because neither device sufficiently restricts forearm supination or pronation, the examiner must emphasize the restriction of turning of door handles, keys, and so forth.
4. Begin *gripping exercises* at half tension after the immobilization phase. Begin with a half grip—just enough to firm the forearm muscles—and gradually build up over 1 to 2 weeks.
5. With restoration of normal grip strength, *isometric toning exercises of wrist flexion* are begun at low tension and slowly increased. The patient should exercise only to the edge of discomfort; patients experiencing forearm muscle soreness are probably exercising too aggressively. Exercises must be interrupted if the medial epicondyle becomes progressively more irritated.
6. The *injection* can be repeated at 6 weeks if improvement in pain, tenderness, or strength is less than 50% and especially if the recovery exercises above are poorly tolerated.
7. *Regular activities, work, and sports* must be delayed until the pain and inflammation have resolved and grip and wrist flexion strength have increased substantially.
8. Long-term recommendations emphasize the need to perform two-handed lifting; a wrist bar when typing; thick, padded grips for tools; and any other changes that would lessen the direct traction or direct pressure on the inner elbow tendons.
9. Obtain *plain film radiographs* of the elbow and consider a *consultation with a surgical orthopedist* for patients with chronic symptoms.

OUTCOME AND FURTHER WORK-UP: Ninety-five percent of patients respond to a combination of rest and restricted use, wrist immobilization, and corticosteroid injection. The remaining 5% may respond to long-term physical therapy toning exercises with severe restrictions of forearm use. Patients failing to restore forearm and wrist function (chronic tendinitis—mucinoid degeneration of the tendon) can be considered for surgical exploration and tendon repair.

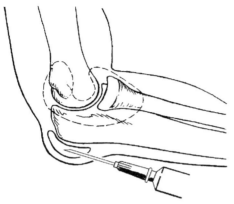

Enter at the base of the bursa
paralleling the ulna; rotate the bevel
so that it faces the bone; aspirate
the entire contents either with the
syringe or with manual pressure;
send for fluid studies
Needle: $1^{1}/_{2}$-inch, 18-gauge
Depth: $^{1}/_{4}$ to $^{3}/_{8}$ inch
Volume: 0.5 mL anesthetic (only in the
dermis) and 0.5 mL K40
NOTE: Apply a compression dressing
with gauze and Coban tape for 24
to 36 hours followed by a protective
neoprene pull-on elbow sleeve for
3 weeks

Figure 3-4A   Aspiration and injection of the olecranon bursa.

SUMMARY

Olecranon bursitis is an inflammation of the bursal sac located between the olecranon process of the ulna and the overlying skin. It is a low-pressure bursa that is susceptible to external pressure. The majority of cases (90%) are caused by repetitive trauma in the form of pressure, commonly referred to as draftsman's elbow. It is one of two bursal sacs that are uniquely susceptible to infection (5% are caused by *Staphylococcus aureus* infection). The remaining 5% of cases are caused by gout. All bursal sacs should be aspirated at presentation in order to define the exact etiology. Septic bursitis should be treated with oral antibiotics and repeated aspiration until clear. Intravenous antibiotics are indicated if cellulitis in the surrounding skin accompanies the bursal infection. Nonseptic bursitis can be treated with the combination of following treatments.

TREATMENT OF CHOICE: Aspiration, drainage, and laboratory analysis are necessary to define the exact etiology.

SEQUENCE OF TREATMENTS

1. Ice applied over the olecranon process is effective in reducing pain and inflammation.
2. Aspiration, drainage, and laboratory analysis (cell count, differential, crystals, Gram stain, and culture) should be performed in every case to define the exact etiology.
3. Following complete drainage, a compression dressing is left in place for 24 to 36 hours.
4. *Acute restriction:* Direct pressure over the olecranon must be avoided for the next 4 weeks.
5. *Most common immobilizer:* A solid, $^{1}/_{4}$-inch-thick neoprene pull-on elbow sleeve should be placed immediately following the compression dressing.
6. *Injection:* Repeat aspiration and injection with triamcinolone acetonide 40 mg/mL (K40) (see page 50) is necessary if the bursa reaccumulates fluid in the first 3 to 4 weeks.
7. *Recovery exercise:* Passive stretching of the elbow in flexion and extension is performed in the uncommon event that the range of motion of the elbow had been reduced.

SURGICAL PROCEDURE: Bursectomy can be considered for persistent swelling or chronic bursal thickening that fails to improve with the combination of aspiration, drainage, and injection of K40 on two successive attempts.

INJECTION: Local injection with corticosteroids is indicated when initial management with simple aspiration followed by compression dressing fails to control swelling and the secondary thickening.

Positioning: The patient is placed in the supine position, the elbow is flexed to 90 degrees, and the arm is placed over the chest.

Surface Anatomy and Point of Entry: The bursal swelling is located directly over the olecranon process. The point of entry is at the base of the bursa along the ulna.

Angle of Entry and Depth: The angle of entry is parallel to the ulna. The depth of the bursa averages between $\frac{1}{4}$ and $\frac{3}{8}$ inch from the surface.

Anesthesia: Ethyl chloride is sprayed on the skin. Local anesthetic is placed in the subcutaneous tissue only (0.5 mL), adjacent to the bursal wall. Intrabursal anesthesia is not necessary because the bursal wall has little in the way of pain receptors.

Technique: In order to avoid recurrent bursal swelling or chronic thickening of the bursal wall, an accurate diagnosis must be made in a timely manner, the inflammatory response must be completely controlled, and the bursa must be protected from further irritation. After the subcutaneous tissue has been anesthetized, an 18-gauge needle is passed, bevel outward, into center of the bursal sac. The bevel is then rotated 180 degrees toward the ulna. Using a combination of aspiration suction and manual compression (milking the fluid with finger pressure on either side), complete decompression of the contents of the bursal sac is accomplished. If infection is suspected, the needle is withdrawn, immediate pressure is applied to avoid any postprocedure bleeding, a compression bandage is applied, and the fluid is sent for studies. For aseptic bursitis—sepsis excluded by lack of fever, risk factors for infection, and so on, clear

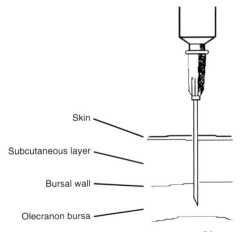

Skin

Subcutaneous layer

Bursal wall

Olecranon bursa

Figure 3-4B   Olecranon bursa aspiration.

acellular serous fluid, and a negative Gram stain—the needle is left in place and the bursa is injected with 0.5 mL of K40 through the same needle. Subsequently, the needle is withdrawn, immediate pressure is applied to avoid any postprocedure bleeding, a compression bandage is applied, and the fluid is sent for studies.

INJECTION AFTERCARE

1. The elbow must be *protected for the first 3 days.* The bulky compression dressing should be left in place for the first 24 to 36 hours and direct pressure and the extremes of range of motion of the elbow must be completely avoided.
2. *Ice* (15 minutes every 4 to 6 hours), *acetaminophen* (1000 mg twice a day), or both, are used for postinjection soreness.
3. The elbow must be *protected for 3 to 4 weeks* with a pull-on neoprene elbow sleeve, worn continuously.
4. Daily passive flexion and extension *stretching exercises* are performed over several weeks if range of motion has been affected (seen exclusively with septic bursitis accompanied by cellulitis).
5. Septic bursitis may require *repeated drainage* at 7- to 10-day intervals.
6. *Injection* with corticosteroids may need to be repeated at 6 weeks if swelling persists or chronic thickening develops. Patient may state, "It feels like I have gravel under my skin!"
7. Direct pressure must be avoided for the next 6 to 12 months.
8. *Consultation:* Bursectomy is considered if the bursa continues to reaccumulate fluid or if chronic thickening of the bursal wall develops (typically bursal wall thickening will undergo a natural involution over the course of 6 months).

OUTCOME AND FURTHER WORK-UP: The success of treatment depends on an accurate diagnosis, appropriate therapy based on laboratory study, complete aspiration of the contents of the bursa, and the padding of the elbow to prevent recurrence. However, even despite these measures, 5% of patients will develop recurrent swelling and thickening of the bursal walls. These cases of chronic bursitis are treated with surgical bursectomy.

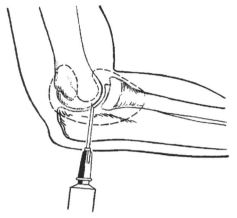

With the elbow flexed to 90 degrees, enter laterally in the center of the triangle formed by the lateral epicondyle, radial head, and olecranon process (typically the center of lateral bulge); the needle should parallel the radial head
Needle: 1-inch, 21- to 22-gauge
Depth: $\frac{5}{8}$ to $\frac{3}{4}$ inch down to and through the radial collateral ligament
Volume: 1 to 2 mL anesthetic and 0.5 mL K40
NOTE: Redirect the needle if bone is encountered at a superficial depth (at $\frac{3}{8}$ inch)

Figure 3-5A   Aspiration and injection of the elbow.

SUMMARY

Aspiration of the radiohumeral joint and synovial analysis are necessary to differentiate the four types of elbow effusion: hemarthrosis, inflammatory, noninflammatory, and septic (see the synovial fluid analysis table, page 210). Rheumatoid arthritis, osteoarthritis due to remote trauma, and spondyloarthropathy with peripheral joint involvement are the most common rheumatic conditions associated with an effusion of the elbow.

TREATMENT OF CHOICE: Because the treatment of choice depends solely on the etiology of the effusion, the first priority is to aspirate synovial fluid for laboratory analysis. Hemarthrosis simply requires drainage. Nonseptic effusions can be treated with corticosteroid injection. Septic arthritis requires immediate institution of parenteral antibiotics. Fortunately, infection of the joint is rare.

SEQUENCE OF TREATMENTS

1. Ice needs to be applied over the entire joint.
2. *Injection:* Aspiration and fluid analysis (cell count, differential, crystals, Gram stain, culture and sensitivity [C/S]) must be performed in order to determine the appropriate set of treatments.
3. *Acute restrictions:* Restricting the extremes of flexion and extension must be balanced against need to maintain range of motion.
4. *Most common immobilizer:* Although not commonly used and obviously a risk factor in developing joint stiffness, a long arm posterior plaster splint can provide temporary supports to the joint.
5. An NSAID in full dose can be used for 2 to 3 weeks but only for the nonseptic effusion (rheumatoid, osteoarthritic, or spondyloarthritic diagnoses).
6. *Injection:* The response to treatment of the nonseptic effusion with local corticosteroid injection is much more predictable than with the NSAID (see page 53).

7. ***Recovery exercise:*** Passive stretching of the elbow in flexion and extension is used to restore any lost range of motion.
8. ***Consultation:*** Surgical consultation is reserved for patients with persistent swelling, loss of smooth motion of the joint, and persistent loss of range of motion.

SURGICAL PROCEDURE: Arthroscopy is used to evaluate for intra-articular loose bodies, osteochondritis dissecans, or for débridement of the osteoarthritic joint.

INJECTION: Aspiration and drainage should be considered for tense, painful hemarthrosis. Corticosteroid injection is indicated for any inflammatory condition that is characterized by a persistent loss of 15 to 20 degrees of extension, flexion, or both, and that has failed to respond to systemic therapy.

Positioning: The patient is placed in the supine position, the elbow is flexed to 90 degrees, and the arm is placed over the chest.
Surface Anatomy and Point of Entry: Joint swelling is most readily seen between the radial head, the olecranon process, and the lateral epicondyle when the elbow is flexed to 90 degrees (the bulge sign of an elbow effusion). The point of entry is at the center of the triangle formed by these three bony prominences.
Angle of Entry and Depth: The angle of entry is perpendicular to the skin, paralleling the radial head. The synovial cavity depth is $\frac{3}{4}$ inch.

Anesthesia: Ethyl chloride is sprayed on the skin. Local anesthetic is placed in the subcutaneous tissue (0.25 mL), in the hard resistance of any bony prominence encountered at a superficial depth (0.25 mL), and at the firm resistance of the deep ligaments (0.25 mL).
Technique: Successful aspiration and drainage require accurate identification of the point of entry and the careful insertion of the needle into the synovial cavity located at the apex of the "inverted cone" formed by the olecranon, lateral epicondyle, and radial head. A **lateral approach** provides the easiest access. A 21- or 22-gauge needle is gently advanced down to the firm resistance of the

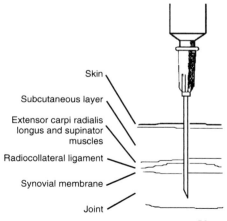

Skin

Subcutaneous layer

Extensor carpi radialis longus and supinator muscles

Radiocollateral ligament

Synovial membrane

Joint

Figure 3-5B   Radiohumeral joint aspiration.

radial collateral ligament, paralleling the radial head. Note: If bone is encountered prematurely at a superficial level ($\frac{3}{8}$ inch), local anesthetic is injected, and the needle is withdrawn $\frac{1}{4}$ inch and redirected. The synovial cavity is at least $\frac{3}{4}$ to 1 inch from the surface! The needle is advanced farther to the radial collateral ligament, another $\frac{1}{4}$ inch through the firm resistance of the ligament to and through the joint capsule. Aspiration is attempted at this depth. If fluid is not readily obtained at this site, the bevel of the needle is rotated 180 degrees and aspiration is attempted again. For the aseptic effusion, the needle is left in place and the joint is injected with 0.5 mL of K40.

INJECTION AFTERCARE

1. All repetitious motion and tension at the elbow must be *avoided for the first 3 days.*
2. *Ice* (15 minutes every 4 to 6 hours), *acetaminophen* (1000 mg twice a day), or both, are used for postinjection soreness.
3. The elbow motion must be *restricted for 3 to 4 weeks* with a pull-on neoprene elbow sleeve, worn continuously.
4. Passive flexion or extension *stretching exercises* are begun as soon as the pain and swelling have abated.
5. Fluid reaccumulation in septic arthritis may need to be *aspirated* again at 7 to 10 days.
6. For nonseptic inflammatory effusions, corticosteroid *injection* may need to be repeated at 6 weeks, especially if swelling persists or chronic synovial thickening develops.
7. *MRI* and a *consultation* with a surgical orthopedist are indicated if signs of osteochondritis dissecans or loose body are present (loss of smooth motion, persistent swelling).

Chapter 4

WRIST

THE DIFFERENTIAL DIAGNOSIS OF WRIST PAIN

DIAGNOSES	CONFIRMATIONS
Wrist pain (most common)	
Simple wrist sprain (ligamentous)	Examination; normal radiographs
Sprain with chondral fracture	Persistent loss of grip, decreased range of motion, and persistent tenderness
Navicular fracture	Loss of 45% of the range of motion; sequential radiographs; plus bone scan
Perilunate dislocation	Loss of the normal bony alignment
Kienböck's disease	Avascular necrosis of the lunate on serial radiographs of the wrist
Triangular cartilage fracture of the ulnocarpal joint	Magnetic resonance imaging (MRI) or arthroscopy
Dorsal ganglion	
From the radiocarpal joint	Aspiration
From the tenosynovial sheath	Aspiration
Carpal tunnel syndrome (CTS)	Nerve conduction velocity testing or local anesthetic block
De Quervain's tenosynovitis	Local anesthetic block
Radiocarpal arthritis	
Post-traumatic osteoarthritis	Radiographs: wrist series
Rheumatoid arthritis	Synovial fluid analysis; erythrocyte sedimentation rate; rheumatoid factor
Gout or pseudogout	Crystal analysis
Referred pain to the wrist	
Carpometacarpal osteoarthritis	Radiographs: thumb series
Cervical spine	Neck rotation; radiograph; MRI
Pronator teres syndrome (mimicking CTS)	Nerve conduction velocity testing

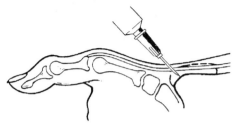

Enter $^3/_8$ inch proximal to the tip of the radial styloid, angling at 45 degrees to the bone, approaching the bone very carefully because of its sensitivity
Needle: $^5/_8$-inch, 25-gauge
Depth: $^3/_8$ to $^1/_2$ inch flush against the periosteum of the radial styloid
Volume: 2 to 3 mL anesthetic and 0.5 mL D80
NOTE: The injection should form a palpable "bubble," $1^1/_2$ inches long

Figure 4-1A   Injection and dilation of de Quervain's tenosynovitis.

SUMMARY

De Quervain's tenosynovitis is an inflammation of the extensor and abductor tendons of the thumb. Repetitive or unaccustomed use of the thumb (gripping and grasping) leads to friction and irritation of the snuff box tendons as they cross the distal radius. Twenty percent of cases occur in young mothers in the first 6 months after delivery (typically from repetitious and unaccustomed lifting of the newborn but occasionally from inappropriate intravenous line placement).

TREATMENT OF CHOICE: A corticosteroid injection properly placed at the radial styloid effectively controls the pain and inflammation in 90% of cases.

SEQUENCE OF TREATMENTS

1. Ice placed over the distal radius is effective in controlling the pain and swelling of mild cases.
2. *Acute restrictions:* Gripping and grasping, especially during the act of lifting, must be restricted.
3. *Most common immobilizer:* A dorsal hood splint or a thumb spica splint is effective if symptoms have been present for less than 6 weeks.
4. *Injection:* The response to corticosteroid injection with depot methylprednisolone 80 mg/mL (D80) is highly efficacious and is indicated if symptoms have been present for longer than 6 weeks (see page 57).
5. *Recovery exercises:* Passively performed stretching of the thumb in flexion is indicated if thumb flexibility has been impaired.
6. *Consultation:* Surgical release can be considered if two injections fail to control the active inflammation.

SURGICAL PROCEDURE: Release of the first dorsal compartment is the procedure of choice if two injections within a year fail to resolve the condition.

INJECTION: Corticosteroid injection is the treatment of choice for patients experiencing symptoms longer than 6 weeks.

Positioning: The wrist is kept in neutral position and turned on its side, radial side up.
Surface Anatomy and Point of Entry: The radial styloid is identified and marked. The point of entry is halfway between the abductor pollicis longus and the extensor pollicis longus tendons as they course over the radial styloid.

Angle of Entry and Depth: The needle is carefully advanced at a 45-degree angle down to the hard resistance of the radial styloid periosteum (pain). If the bone is not encountered at $\frac{3}{8}$ to $\frac{1}{2}$ inch (typical depth), the point of entry may have been too distal!

Anesthesia: Ethyl chloride is sprayed on the skin. Local anesthetic is placed just above at the radius.

Technique: Successful treatment involves a single passage of the needle down to the periosteum of the radius, slow dilation of the tissues with anesthetic, and injection with D80 all in one step. After freezing the skin with ethyl chloride spray, a 25-gauge needle is gently advanced down to the radial styloid and 2 to 2.5 mL of anesthesia is slowly injected, allowing the soft tissues to gradually dilate over the tendons (a bubble should appear). Moderate pressure to injection, a poorly distensible sac, or both may indicate a chronic stenosis of the tendons, that is, adhesions. With the needle left in place (avoid multiple punctures!), the syringe containing the anesthetic is removed and replaced with the syringe containing 0.5 mL of D80. The treatment is competed by injecting the corticosteroid.

INJECTION AFTERCARE
1. The area must be ***protected for first 3 days*** by avoiding all gripping, grasping, and direct pressure.
2. ***Ice*** (15 minutes every 4 to 6 hours), ***acetaminophen (Tylenol ES)*** (1000 mg twice a day), or both, are used for postinjection soreness.
3. The wrist motion must be ***restricted for 3 to 4 weeks*** with a dorsal hood splint, a thumb spica splint, or a Velcro wrist immobilizer worn during the day (optional).
4. Begin passive ***stretching exercises*** of the thumb in flexion at 3 weeks.
5. The ***injection*** can be repeated at 6 weeks if symptoms have not improved by 50% (warning: skin and subcutaneous fat atrophy may be greater or permanent with a second injection—30%).
6. In order to avoid recurrence, the need to avoid grasping and lifting with the wrist ulnar deviated is emphasized again.

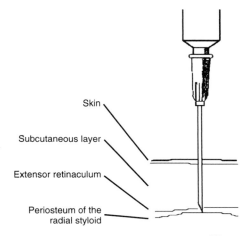

Skin

Subcutaneous layer

Extensor retinaculum

Periosteum of the radial styloid

Figure 4-1B De Quervain's tenosynovitis.

7. A *consultation* with a surgical orthopedist is considered if two injections in 1 year fail to resolve the condition.

OUTCOME AND FURTHER WORK-UP: Corticosteroid injection effectively resolves this classic inflammatory tenosynovitis. Radiographs of the wrist are usually not necessary except in the case of tenosynovitis accompanied by arthritis of the wrist or carpometacarpal joint. Nerve conduction velocity testing is necessary when hypoesthesias or paresthesia accompany the condition; direct involvement of the radial nerve or concomitant carpal tunnel can occur with de Quervain's tenosynovitis.

RESULTS: These data were published July 1991 by Anderson and colleagues (Table 4-1).

Table 4-1   Clinical Outcomes of 55 Cases of De Quervain's Tenosynovitis Treated with Depo-Medrol 80 mg/mL (4.2-Year Prospective Follow-up of 95% of Patients Enrolled)

Complete resolution (single injection)	30 (58%)
Recurrence (reinjected—average 11.9 months to recurrence)	17 (32%)
Failed to respond; chronic tendinitis	5 (10%)
TOTAL	52

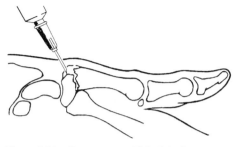

Enter $^3/_8$ inch proximal to the base of the metacarpal bone, in the anatomic "snuff box," adjacent to the abductor pollicis longus tendon
Needle: $^5/_8$-inch, 25-gauge
Depth: $^1/_2$ to $^5/_8$ inch flush against the trapezium bone
Volume: 0.5 mL anesthetic injected at $^3/_8$ inch and 0.5 mL K40 injected flush against the trapezium
NOTE: Moderate pressure may be necessary

Figure 4-2A   Carpometacarpal joint injection.

SUMMARY

Carpometacarpal (CMC) joint arthritis is a "wear-and-tear" arthritis of the base of the thumb. Pain, swelling, and bony deformity occur at the articulation between the metacarpal bone and the trapezium. Advanced disease is associated with loss of articular cartilage, osteophyte formation, and subluxation of the metacarpal bone. Although this is a common form of osteoarthritis, it does not herald the onset of systemic forms of osteoarthritis.

TREATMENT OF CHOICE: Corticosteroid injection placed deep in the anatomic snuff box is effective for all stages of the condition.

SEQUENCE OF TREATMENTS

1.   Ice is applied over the base of the thumb,
2.   *Acute restrictions:* Gripping and grasping must be restricted during treatment and altered to prevent future arthritic flare-ups.
3.   *Most common immobilizer:* Immobilization with overlap-taping of the joint, a thumb spica splint, or a dorsal hood splint is the preferred treatment in the first 6 weeks of a flare-up.
4.   *Injection:* Corticosteroid injection with triamcinolone acetonide 40 mg/mL (K40) is indicated if symptoms have been present for longer than 6 weeks (see page 60).
5.   *Recovery exercises:* After the acute symptoms have been controlled, stretching exercises of thumb in flexion and extension are used to restore the range of motion followed by active gripping exercises to improve strength.
6.   *Consultation:* Surgical consultation can be considered if two injections, fixed immobilization, and physical therapy exercises fail to restore the function of the thumb and hand.

SURGICAL PROCEDURE: Tendon interpositional arthroplasty (the use of the flexor carpi radialis tendon as a spacer between the trapezium and the proximal metacarpal) and trapezial arthroplasty (replacement of the trapezium bone) are the two most commonly performed procedures. Either procedure is effective in controlling the symptoms of the arthritic flare and restoring at least a portion of the patient's function.

INJECTION: Local anesthetic injection is used to differentiate CMC arthritis from de Quervain's tenosynovitis or wrist arthritis. Corticosteroid injection is the anti-inflammatory treatment of choice for symptoms persisting beyond 8 weeks.

Positioning: The wrist is placed in neutral position with the radial side turned up.

Surface Anatomy and Point of Entry: The proximal end of the metacarpal bone is identified and marked. The point of entry is $\frac{3}{8}$ inch proximal to the metacarpal and adjacent to the abductor pollicis longus tendon.

Angle of Entry and Depth: The needle is carefully advanced at a 45-degree angle down to the hard resistance of the trapezium (typical depth is $\frac{1}{2}$ to $\frac{5}{8}$ inch).

Anesthesia: Ethyl chloride is sprayed on the skin. Local anesthetic is placed in the subcutaneous fat (0.5 mL) and $\frac{1}{4}$ inch above the trapezium (0.5 mL).

Technique: The successful injection must be placed in the depths of the snuff box and at the level of the periosteum of the trapezium! After placing anesthetic in the superficial layers, the needle is gently advanced at a 45-degree angle down to the trapezium bone ($\frac{1}{2}$ to $\frac{5}{8}$ inch). If the hard resistance of bone is encountered at a superficial depth ($\frac{3}{8}$ inch), the needle is withdrawn and redirected (this is usually the case when the point of entry is too distal—a common error). Note: Anesthetic should be placed just above the trapezium bone, reserving the deeper site for the corticosteroid. The radial artery courses through the snuff box. If the needle is advanced slowly, the artery will move to the side. However, if the artery is encountered (blood immediately entering the syringe), withdraw completely out of the skin, hold pressure for 5 minutes, and reenter $\frac{1}{4}$ inch to either side.

INJECTION AFTERCARE
1. The thumb and wrist must be ***protected for the first 3 days*** by avoiding all grasping, pinching, vibration, and direct pressure.
2. ***Ice*** (15 minutes every 4 to 6 hours), ***acetaminophen*** (1000 mg twice a day), or both, are used for postinjection soreness.

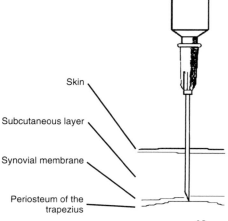

Skin

Subcutaneous layer

Synovial membrane

Periosteum of the trapezius

Figure 4-2B   Carpometacarpal joint injection.

60

3. The thumb motion must be *restricted for 3 to 4 weeks* by limiting grasping, pinching, and exposure to vibration or for greater protection with overlap-taping the joint, a dorsal hood splint, or a thumb spica splint.
4. Practical recommendations are emphasized, including light gripping of the pen, padding of hand tools, antivibration gloves, oversized grips for sports equipment (golf clubs, rackets, etc.) and so forth.
5. Passive *stretching exercises* of the thumb in flexion and extension are recommended if the range of motion was impaired either by the condition or because of the immobilization.
6. The *injection* can be repeated at 6 weeks if symptoms have not improved by 50%.
7. A *consultation* with a surgical orthopedist can be considered if two injections, immobilization, and physical therapy fail to improve thumb and hand function continuously over 3 to 4 months.

OUTCOME AND FURTHER WORK-UP: CMC osteoarthritis predictably responds to corticosteroid injection. Mild wear-and-tear treated with injection may be arrested for years until a subsequent injury or overuse causes an arthritic flare-up. However, remission after injection gradually shortens with progressive loss of cartilage, bony enlargement, and subluxation. When injection fails to provide months of relief, surgical intervention can be entertained.

RESULTS: These data were generated at the Sunnyside Medical Orthopedic Clinic 1990 to 1996 (Table 4-2).

Table 4-2 Clinical Outcomes of 50 Cases of Carpometacarpal Osteoarthritis Treated with Kenalog 40 mg/mL

Epidemiology: Average age—50 years (range 34-83); ratio of women to men—7:1; right side was equally affected as left side

Injection results: 46 of 50 (92%) responded to single or multiple treatment, averaging 10 months of relief (range 3-19 months)

Surgery: Four patients failed to respond and underwent surgery

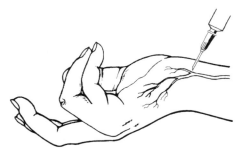

Enter $^1/_2$ to $^3/_4$ inch proximal to the palmar prominence of the wrist, at the distal volar crease, and on the ulnar side of palmaris longus tendon (there is a greater space between the palmaris longus tendon and the pisiform bone!)
Needle: $^5/_8$-inch, 25-gauge
Depth: $^1/_2$ to $^5/_8$ inch
Volume: 1 to 2 mL anesthetic and 0.5 mL K40
NOTE: If the patient experiences nerve irritation, withdraw 1 or 2 mm or redirect to the radial or ulnar side

Figure 4-3A   Carpal tunnel injection.

SUMMARY

CTS is a compression neuropathy of the median nerve. Compression occurs under the transverse carpal ligament at the wrist, at the pronator teres muscle in the proximal forearm, or rarely, in the distal forearm following penetrating trauma. Patients present with a variety of symptoms including hypoesthesias, dysesthetic pain in the forearm and hand, muscle weakness, or motor loss with atrophy. Advanced CTS with motor involvement should be treated with surgical release. Mild to moderate CTS (sensory symptoms only) can be managed with a combination of medical treatments.

TREATMENT OF CHOICE: The treatment of choice depends on the stage of the condition. Ergonomic adjustments at the work station and wrist splinting are the treatments of choice at the time of initial presentation.

SEQUENCE OF TREATMENTS

1. *Acute restrictions:* Gripping, grasping, and repetitive use of the wrist must be reduced.
2. Ergonomic adjustments at the work station are necessary acutely and over the long term.
3. *Most common immobilizer:* A Velcro wrist immobilizer with metal stay is used to reduce the symptoms manifesting at night, but may need to be used continuously, day and night, for optimal results.
4. *Exercise of choice:* Gentle stretching exercises of the finger flexors in extension is recommended.
5. Approximately 20% of patients respond to a 2- to 3-week trial of an oral diuretic when manifesting significant fluid retention (tight rings, ankle edema, bloating, and so forth).
6. Nerve conduction velocity (NCV) testing is advised for patients with persistent or progressive symptoms, patients with motor involvement (subjective weakness, diminished grip strength, atrophy), and patients contemplating surgery.
7. *Injection:* Corticosteroid injection with K40 is appropriate for patients experiencing sensory symptoms only (see page 63).
8. Corticosteroid injection can be repeated if symptoms have not improved by 50%.
9. *Recovery exercise:* Extension stretching exercises of the eight flexor tendons of the fingers maintains hand flexibility and theoretically diminishes the pressure on the nerve.

10. **Consultation:** Consultation with a neurosurgeon or orthopedic surgeon is considered if two injections fail to control sensory symptoms and strongly advised if the patient demonstrates impairment or loss of motor function.

SURGICAL PROCEDURE: Release of the transverse carpal ligament reduces the pressure on the median nerve and is indicated for either persistent symptoms or motor involvement (recurrent median nerve involvement).

INJECTION: Injection with corticosteroids can be used for definitive treatment of mild to moderate sensory CTS, or a positive response to injection can be used as an aid in the diagnosis of mild CTS with normal NCV testing. Approximately 30% of patients with CTS have intermittent symptoms, equivocal signs on examination of the upper extremity and neck, and normal NCV testing. Because patients with this constellation of findings still respond to corticosteroid injection (90%), empiric treatment has been advocated as a diagnostic aid.

Positioning: The wrist is positioned palm up and dorsiflexed to 30 degrees (see Fig. 4-3A).

Surface Anatomy and Point of Entry: The pisiform bone and the palmaris longus tendons are located and marked. The point of entry is at the intersection of the distal volar crease and the ulnar side of palmaris longus.

Angle of Entry and Depth: The needle is carefully advanced at a 45-degree angle down to and through the transverse carpal ligament (typical depth is $\frac{3}{8}$ to $\frac{1}{2}$ inch). This angle coupled with the short $\frac{5}{8}$-inch needle makes it nearly impossible to enter the nerve!

Anesthesia: Ethyl chloride is sprayed on the skin. Local anesthetic is placed in the subcutaneous fat (0.5 mL), at the firm resistance of the transverse carpal ligament (0.5 mL), and in the carpal tunnel (0.5 to 1 mL). Anesthesia in the distribution of the median nerve confirms the accurate placement.

Technique: The successful injection of the carpal tunnel requires medication placement just below the transverse carpal ligament. The proper depth can be determined by measurement, feel as the

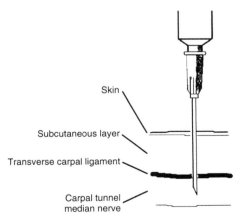

Skin

Subcutaneous layer

Transverse carpal ligament

Carpal tunnel
median nerve

Figure 4-3B   Carpal tunnel injection.

needle is advanced, and the flow of medication. Based on the point of entry and the 45-degree angle of entry, the proper depth of injection is $\frac{1}{2}$ to $\frac{5}{8}$ inch. As the needle is advanced through the tissues, a pop or "giving way" sensation is often felt as soon as the needle passes through the ligament and into the tunnel. Lastly, the flow of medication above the transverse ligament requires moderate pressure as opposed to the minimum pressure that is required when injecting medication in the tunnel! The patient may experience a temporary median nerve irritation when the needle enters the tunnel. Note: If the patient continues to feel nerve irritation with injection, either reposition the needle or withdraw $\frac{1}{8}$ inch.

INJECTION AFTERCARE
1. The wrist must be *protected for the first 3 days* by avoiding all wrist movement, finger motion, vibration exposure, and direct pressure.
2. *Ice* (15 minutes every 4 to 6 hours), *acetaminophen* (1000 mg twice a day), or both, are used for postinjection soreness.
3. The wrist motion must be *limited for 3 to 4 weeks* by limiting grasping, pinching, and vibration exposure and by wearing a Velcro wrist immobilizer with metal stay.
4. The need to make ergonomic adjustments at the work station is constantly reevaluated.
5. Begin passive *stretching exercises* of the fingers in extension at 3 to 4 weeks.
6. The *injection* can be repeated at 6 weeks if symptoms have not improved by 50%.
7. *Consultation* with a neurosurgeon or surgical orthopedist can be considered if two injections fail to provide at least 4 to 6 months of symptomatic relief and is mandatory if motor function begins to fail.

OUTCOME AND FURTHER WORK-UP: Progressive sensory or advanced sensorimotor form of carpal tunnel should be treated surgically to avoid permanent nerve injury. The use of corticosteroid injection should be limited to patients desiring a temporary control of mild, intermittent sensory symptoms.

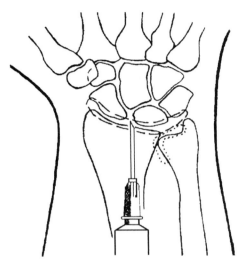

Enter the joint between the junction of the distal radius, the navicular, and the lunate bones located at the intersection of the distal radius and the radial side of the extensor tendon of the index finger
Needle: $^{5}/_{8}$-inch, 25-gauge for anesthetic and injection; 21-gauge for aspiration
Depth: A depth of $^{1}/_{2}$ inch ensures an intra-articular injection
Volume: 1 mL anesthetic and 0.5 mL K40
NOTE: If the hard resistance of bone is encountered at $^{1}/_{4}$ inch, then withdraw through the radionavicular ligaments, use skin traction to redirect the needle, and advance the needle into the joint

Figure 4-4A   Dorsal approach to arthrocentesis and injection of the wrist joint.

SUMMARY
Aspiration of synovial fluid and laboratory analysis are indicated to differentiate post-traumatic monarthritis, crystal-induced arthropathy, rheumatoid arthritis, and the uncommon septic arthritis. Radiocarpal joint involvement in rheumatoid arthritis is very common. Osteoarthritis of the wrist is uncommon and nearly always results from injury (multiple wrist sprains, fracture of the navicular or distal radius, or dislocation of the carpal bones). Significant swelling of the wrist joint is nearly always associated with loss of flexion and extension (normal range of motion in flexion is 90 degrees and 80 degrees in extension on average).

TREATMENT OF CHOICE: Aspiration and synovial fluid analysis (see synovial fluid analysis table on page 210) are mandatory to define the exact etiology. Corticosteroid injection is the treatment of choice for the inflammatory, nonseptic effusion.

SEQUENCE OF TREATMENTS
1. Ice is placed over the dorsum of the wrist.
2. *Acute restrictions:* Gripping, grasping, and repetitive use of the wrist are restricted.
3. Ergonomic adjustments at the work station can include keeping repetitive work within 1 to $1^{1}/_{2}$ feet of the torso, keeping the wrists straight and aligned with the forearms, and performing the majority of lifting with both hands.
4. *Most common immobilizer:* A Velcro wrist immobilizer with metal stay guarantees the wrist is well supported and kept straight, aligned with the forearms.

5. ***Exercises of choice:*** Gentle stretching exercises of wrist flexion and extension are prescribed if range of motion has been impaired.
6. A 2- to 3-week trial of an oral nonsteroidal anti-inflammatory drug (NSAID) in full dosage is prescribed for mild to moderate symptoms that have been present for just a few weeks.
7. ***Injection:*** If symptoms are moderate to severe or chronic (present for weeks), an intra-articular injection with K40 is indicated (see pages 66-67).
8. ***Consultation:*** Orthopedic consultation can be considered if two injections and immobilization fail to control symptoms and examination demonstrates at least a 50% impairment of the range of motion.

SURGICAL PROCEDURE: Arthrodesis (fusion) of the wrist is the procedure of choice for severe arthritis.

INJECTION: Local corticosteroid injection is commonly used when ice, restricted use, immobilization, and an oral NSAID fail to control symptoms.

Positioning: The hand and wrist are placed in the prone position. The wrist is flexed to 30 degrees and held in place with a rolled-up towel, placed under the wrist.

Surface Anatomy and Point of Entry: The extensor tendon of the index finger is identified and marked as it crosses the radius. The very edge of the distal radius is palpated and marked. The point of entry is on the radial side of the intersection of the tendon and the distal edge of the radius. Alternatively, the exact point of entry can be found by gently placing a pen firmly against the skin between the radius, navicular, and lunate. The point of entry is determined where the pen makes the greatest indentation.

Angle of Entry and Depth: The needle is inserted perpendicular to the skin. If the firm resistance of bone or ligament is encountered at a superficial depth ($\frac{1}{4}$ to $\frac{3}{8}$ inch), the needle is withdrawn back through the dorsal radionavicular ligament and repositioned with the aid of skin traction. The needle should pass smoothly the $\frac{1}{2}$-inch distance into the joint if the point of entry is correct.

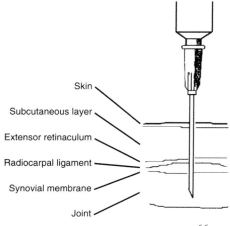

Skin
Subcutaneous layer
Extensor retinaculum
Radiocarpal ligament
Synovial membrane
Joint

Figure 4-4B Radiocarpal joint injection.

Anesthesia: Ethyl chloride is sprayed on the skin. Local anesthetic is placed in the subcutaneous fat (0.5 mL), the firm resistance of the radiocarpal ligament (0.5 mL), and in the joint (0.5 mL).

Technique: The **dorsal approach** is preferred. The successful injection will carefully enter the $\frac{1}{4}$-inch space between the radius, navicular, and lunate at a depth of $\frac{1}{2}$ inch. The 25-gauge needle is advanced perpendicularly through the radionavicular ligament and into the wrist. The needle must be redirected if bone is encountered at $\frac{1}{4}$ inch. If fluid is not obtained with the 25-gauge needle, a 22-gauge needle can be used to aspirate. If aspiration is still negative, the joint can be irrigated with 1 to 2 mL of sterile saline and sent for Gram stain and culture. For the nonseptic effusion, the needle is left in place and the joint is injected with 0.5 mL of K40.

INJECTION AFTERCARE

1. The wrist must be *protected for the first 3 days* by avoiding repetitive motion and tension across the wrist and direct pressure.
2. *Ice* (15 minutes every 4 to 6 hours), *acetaminophen* (1000 mg twice a day), or both, are used for postinjection soreness.
3. The wrist motion must be *restricted for 3 to 4 weeks* with a Velcro wrist brace worn continuously for the first week (especially for advanced disease with loss of 30% to 40% of range of motion).
4. *Isometric toning exercises* of wrist flexion and extension are begun at 3 weeks.
5. The *injection* can be repeated at 6 weeks if swelling persists or chronic synovial thickening (synovitis) develops.
6. Long-term protection of the joint is discussed (avoid vibration exposure and heavy impact, maintain forearm muscle tone to support the joint, wear a wrist brace with heavy use).
7. Obtain a *consultation* with a surgical orthopedist if symptoms persist, 50% of normal range of motion has been lost, and the patient is willing to undergo surgical fusion.

OUTCOME AND FURTHER WORK-UP: To ensure optimal results, corticosteroid injection should be combined with fixed immobilization. Work-up should always include synovial fluid analysis and sent for Gram stain and culture if only a small amount of fluid is obtained. If fluid is not obtained, empiric treatment is based on the clues from the examination; plain film radiographs of the wrist, which are often more helpful in differentiating rheumatoid, osteoarthritic, and crystal-induced arthritis; or MRI to evaluate the integrity of the triangular cartilage of the separate ulnocarpal joint.

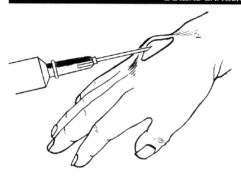

Enter at the base of the palpable cyst, paralleling the skin and avoiding the adjacent veins or tendons
Needle: $^5/_8$-inch, 25-gauge for anesthetic; $1^1/_2$ inches, 18-gauge for aspiration
Depth: Superficial, rarely less than $^3/_8$ inch
Volume: 0.5 mL anesthetic in the subcutaneous tissues adjacent to the cyst wall and 0.5 mL K40
NOTE: A 10-mL syringe is necessary to obtain enough vacuum pressure to aspirate the highly viscous fluid

Figure 4-5A Dorsal ganglion aspiration and injection.

SUMMARY

A dorsal ganglion is an abnormal accumulation of synovial or tenosynovial fluid that has leaked outside the confines of the normal synovial cavity or tenosynovial sheath, causing an inflammatory reaction in the subcutaneous tissue and subsequent cyst wall formation. The overproduction of fluid is always caused by a subtle abnormality of the wrist joint or the extensor tendon sheath (old cartilaginous or tendon injury, poor muscular support, hypermobility because of lax supporting ligaments, etc.). The fluid, rich in protein content, irritates the tissues and leads to cyst formation. Other names for this common condition include Bible cyst, wrist cyst, or dorsal tendon cyst. Volar ganglions—on the palm side of the wrist—are much less common.

TREATMENT OF CHOICE: Many ganglia simply undergo involution over time. Hence treatment can consist of explanation, reassurance, and observation. But some patients request definitive treatment. Simple aspiration of the contents of the cyst is the initial treatment of choice.

SEQUENCE OF TREATMENTS

1. For small ganglia that have been present a few weeks, simple observation is recommended because a proportion will undergo involution.
2. *Acute restrictions:* Encourage restriction of wrist motion, avoidance of vibration, and ergonomic adjustments at the work station (keeping the repetitive work within 1 to $1^1/_2$ feet directly in front, keeping the wrists aligned with the forearms, and performing lifting with both hands).
3. *Most common immobilizer:* The restriction imposed by a Velcro wrist immobilizer with metal stay should reduce the overproduction of fluid.
4. *Injection:* Simple aspiration will resolve at least half since the overproduction is not associated with a chronic or recurrent wrist condition (see details page 69).
5. For recurrent cysts, aspiration can be combined with corticosteroid injection with K40.
6. *Recovery exercises:* Isometric toning exercises of flexion and extension are used when the ganglion is associated with a chronic or recurrent wrist condition.
7. *Consultation:* Orthopedic surgical consultation is considered if the patient has pressure symptoms, radial nerve paresthesias, or chronic wrist condition with significant loss of range of function (motion or strength).

SURGICAL PROCEDURE: Excision of the cyst and sinus tract.

INJECTION: Aspiration is the treatment of choice for ganglia that fail to resolve with time. At least half these will respond to simple aspiration. Corticosteroid injection is the treatment of choice for ganglia that cause pressure on the superficial branches of the radial nerve (dysesthetic pain on the dorsum of the hand and fingers) or for recurrent cysts that are larger than 1 inch in diameter.

Positioning: The hand and wrist are placed in the prone position. The wrist is flexed to 30 to 45 degrees and held in place with a rolled-up towel.

Surface Anatomy and Point of Entry: Most dorsal ganglions are located directly over the navicular bone and are more prominent when the wrist is flexed. The point of entry is at the proximal base of the cyst away from any local vein or tendon.

Angle of Entry and Depth: The 18-gauge needle is advanced into the center of the cyst, paralleling the skin. The depth is rarely more than $\frac{1}{4}$ to $\frac{3}{8}$ inch from the surface.

Anesthesia: Ethyl chloride is sprayed on the skin. Local anesthetic is placed in the subcutaneous fat adjacent to the cyst (the cyst wall has few if any nerve endings).

Technique: Success of injection depends on aspiration of the entire contents of the cyst and subsequent injection of corticosteroid through the same needle. Optimal aspiration is accomplished by entering the **base of the ganglion.** An 18-gauge needle attached to a 10-mL syringe is advanced into the center of the cyst. The bevel of the needle is rotated 180 degrees and the highly viscous fluid is removed. Manual pressure applied from either side may assist in the removal of the fluid. With the needle left in place, the cyst in injected with 0.5 mL of K40.

INJECTION AFTERCARE
1. The wrist must be *protected for the first 3 days* by avoiding repetitive motion and tension across the wrist and direct pressure.

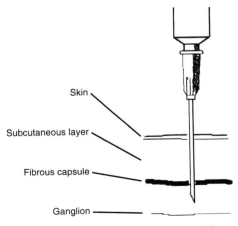

Skin

Subcutaneous layer

Fibrous capsule

Ganglion

Figure 4-5B Dorsal ganglion injection.

2. *Ice* (15 minutes every 4 to 6 hours), *acetaminophen* (1000 mg twice a day), or both, are used for postinjection soreness.
3. The wrist motion must be *restricted for 3 to 4 weeks* by avoiding repetitive lifting, gripping, grasping, and vibration.
4. A Velcro wrist brace is strongly advised if advanced wrist arthritis is present.
5. If the forearm muscles have weakened from disuse, begin *isometric toning exercises* of wrist flexion and extension at 3 weeks.
6. The *injection* can be repeated at 6 weeks with a corticosteroid if fluid reaccumulates.
7. Consider an intra-articular injection of the radiocarpal joint to reduce the overproduction of joint fluid (especially with significant radiocarpal joint disease).
8. Obtain a *consultation* with a surgical orthopedist if the patient has pressure symptoms, radial nerve paresthesias, or swelling that interferes with normal wrist motion.

OUTCOME AND FURTHER WORK-UP: Without exception, patients diagnosed with a dorsal ganglion have an underlying radiocarpal joint or extensor tenosynovitis causing an overproduction of fluid. Work-up may be limited to a thorough examination of the wrist joint, extensor tendons, and measurement of grip and forearm muscle strength, but can include radiographic studies to identify the subtle abnormalities involving the joint or tendons. All patients must be apprised of the relationship of the ganglion to the subtle abnormalities affecting the joint and tendons and the frequent recurrence rates based on this relationship.

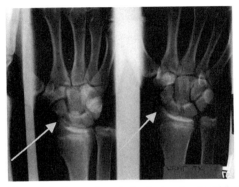

A tentative diagnosis of navicular fracture is made if the patient has sustained a fall to an outstretched hand or has suffered a direct blow to the wrist, especially when associated with the following signs: (1) dramatic tenderness over the dorsum of the wrist, (2) dramatic tenderness in the anatomic snuff box, and (3) loss of half the normal range of motion as a result of pain and mechanical limitation of motion. Treatment of choice: Fixed immobilization to protect against avascular necrosis, nonunion, or medicolegal entanglement!

Figure 4-6 Traumatic navicular fracture (*arrow,* midbody fracture).

SUMMARY

Patients with an uncomplicated sprained wrist can be treated with ice, a simple wrist brace, and limited use over 7 to 10 days with uniformly good results. However, when wrist pain is severe, snuff box or navicular tenderness is dramatic, and the range of motion of the wrist has been decreased by 50%, the health care provider must evaluate and *treat* for navicular fracture, lunate dislocation, or carpal avascular necrosis. Failure to recognize the fracture can result in a poor outcome for the patient and potential medicolegal issues for the health care provider.

TREATMENT OF CHOICE: If navicular fracture is suspected, suggested either by the severity of the injury or the dramatic changes on examination, then fixed immobilization of the wrist and thumb and close follow-up are mandatory! **Medicolegal issue:** Navicular fracture is associated with avascular necrosis and nonunion of the fracture fragments in a small percentage of cases. Because the outcome is so poor with either one of these conditions—chronic wrist pain and poor range of motion—failure to immobilize the wrist and thumb is perceived as malpractice.

SEQUENCE OF TREATMENTS

1. *Plain film radiographs* of the wrist are obtained initially.
2. *Injection:* Local anesthetic block may be necessary to differentiate extensor tenosynovitis or de Quervain's tenosynovitis from involvement of the radionavicular joint (pages 56-57).
3. *Most common immobilizer:* A short arm cast or posterior splint that incorporates immobilization of the thumb is worn continuously until orthopedic surgeon consultation is completed.
4. Radiographs should be repeated at 2 to 4 weeks to evaluate the progress of healing and to exclude avascular necrosis or bony nonunion.
5. *Consultation:* Orthopedic surgical consultation is strongly recommended for any suspected or confirmed case of navicular fracture.

6. ***Recovery exercises:*** Gentle range of motion exercises of the wrist in flexion and extension are begun when radiographic evidence of healing is well under way.

SURGICAL PROCEDURE: Navicular replacement (arthroplasty) and fusion (arthrodesis) are the two most common procedures.

Chapter 5

HAND

THE DIFFERENTIAL DIAGNOSIS OF HAND PAIN

DIAGNOSES	CONFIRMATIONS
Osteoarthritis (most common)	
Heberden's and Bouchard's nodes	Examination; radiographs: hand series
Post-traumatic monarthric osteoarthritis	Examination; radiographs: hand series
Mucinoid cysts atop the joint	Examination; simple puncture
Erosive subtype of osteoarthritis	Radiographs: hand series
Flexor tendons	
Trigger finger/flexor tenosynovitis	Examination
Fixed locked digit	Examination
Tendon cyst	Examination; simple puncture
Benign giant cell tumor	Surgical removal; pathology
Palmar fascia	
Palmar fibromatosis without contracture	Examination
Dupuytren's contracture	Examination
Limited joint mobility syndrome (in long-standing diabetes)	Examination
Extensor tendons	
Mallet finger	Examination
Dorsotenosynovitis	Examination
Reflex sympathetic dystrophy	Examination; bone scan
Rheumatoid arthritis	Synovial fluid analysis; erythrocyte sedimentation rate; rheumatoid factor
Post-traumatic metacarpophalangeal joint arthritis	Examination; local anesthetic block; radiographs
Gamekeeper's thumb	Examination; local anesthetic block

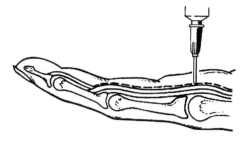

The point of entry for the *finger* is just proximal to the first volar crease in the midline, directly over the center of the tendon. The point of entry for the *thumb* is at the distal volar crease in the midline, directly over the center of the tendon.
Needle: ⅝-inch, 25-gauge
Depth: ¼ to ⅜ inch, flush against the tendon
Volume: 0.5 mL anesthetic and 0.25 mL D80
NOTE: Never inject with hard pressure, intratendinous! If the patient experiences pain, withdraw 1 to 2 mm

Figure 5-1A   Trigger finger injection.

SUMMARY

Trigger finger is an inflammation of the two flexor tendons of the finger as they cross the metacarpophalangeal (MCP) head in the palm. Repetitive gripping and grasping and direct pressure over the MCP joint (tools, golf clubs, etc.) cause swelling of the tendon and inflammation of the tendon sheath (stage 1—active tenosynovitis). As the tendon swelling increases, the two flexor tendons lose their smooth motion through the sheath and under the A-1 pulley ligament, the specialized ligament that anchors the tendons to the metacarpal bone (stage 2—triggering or mechanical catching). If the tendon continues to swell, an irreversible threshold is reached, the tendons can no longer pass under the A-1 pulley, and the finger remains in a locked position (stage 3—fixed locked digit).

TREATMENT OF CHOICE: Buddy-taping is the treatment of choice for symptoms less than 6 weeks in duration and corticosteroid injection for symptoms lasting longer than 6 weeks.

SEQUENCE OF TREATMENTS

1. *Most common immobilization:* Buddy-taping two fingers together is used to reduce movement of the affected finger.
2. *Acute restrictions:* The intensity of gripping, grasping, and pinching must be reduced.
3. *Injection:* Persistent symptoms are treated with corticosteroid injection with depot methylprednisolone 80 mg/mL (D80) at the A-1 pulley (see details on page 75).
4. *Recovery exercise:* Gentle passive stretching in extension is begun once symptoms have improved significantly.
5. Injection is repeated at 5 to 6 weeks if symptoms have not improved dramatically.
6. *Consultation:* Surgical consultation is considered if the mechanical triggering fails to respond to two injections within 12 months or for a fixed locked digit (unable to straighten).

SURGICAL PROCEDURE: Surgical release of the A-1 pulley ligament either percutaneously or by traditional surgical incision are the procedures of choice.

INJECTION: Local injection is the anti-inflammatory treatment of choice, especially if symptoms have been present for more than 6 weeks, simple immobilization has failed, or if the patient presents with severe locking.

Positioning: The hand is positioned flat on the examination table with the palm up and the fingers outstretched.

Surface Anatomy and Point of Entry: The proximal volar crease of the *finger* or the distal volar crease over the MP joint of the *thumb* is identified. The point of entry for the *finger* is just proximal to the first volar crease in the midline. The point of entry for the *thumb* is at the distal volar crease in the midline.

Angle of Entry and Depth: The needle is inserted perpendicular to the skin. The depth of injection is $\frac{1}{4}$ to $\frac{3}{8}$ inch for trigger *finger* and $\frac{1}{8}$ to $\frac{1}{4}$ inch for trigger *thumb*.

Anesthesia: Ethyl chloride is sprayed on the skin. Local anesthetic is placed in the subcutaneous tissue.

Technique: A **volar approach** directly over the center of the tendon is preferred. After applying the ethyl chloride spray, the skin is grasped and pinched up to facilitate the entry of the needle and reduce the chance of inserting the needle directly into the superficially located tendon. Local anesthetic is placed just under the skin. Then the needle is carefully advanced down to the firm resistance of the flexor tendon, a rubbery-like sensation. The needle is held flush against the tendon, using just the weight of the syringe. Without advancing the needle, the corticosteroid is injected just atop the tendon and hence underneath the tenosynovial sheath.

INJECTION AFTERCARE
1. The finger must be ***protected for the first 3 days***, avoiding direct pressure and all gripping and grasping.
2. Buddy tape placed across the adjacent two fingers is used for the first few days.

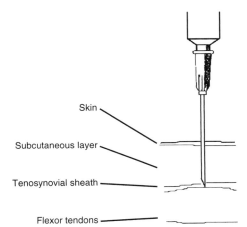

Skin

Subcutaneous layer

Tenosynovial sheath

Flexor tendons

Figure 5-1B   Trigger finger injection.

3. *Ice* (15 minutes every 4 to 6 hours), *acetaminophen (Tylenol ES)* (1000 mg twice a day), or both, are used for postinjection soreness.
4. Use of the fingers should be *limited for 3 to 4 weeks* by avoiding repetitive gripping, grasping, pressure over the MCP heads, and vibration.
5. Passive *stretching exercises* of the fingers in extension are begun at 3 weeks.
6. The *injection* can be repeated at 6 weeks with corticosteroid if tenosynovitis or locking persists.
7. Padded gloves and padded tools are suggested for long-term prevention in recurrent cases.
8. Obtain a *consultation* with a surgical orthopedist if two consecutive injections fail to provide at least 6 months of relief.

OUTCOME AND FURTHER WORK-UP: Local corticosteroid injection is the treatment of choice for trigger finger. Patients with recurrent tenosynovitis or mechanical locking need to evaluate their work and recreation habits to identify activities that cause pressure over the A-1 pulley or those activities that require excessive gripping and grasping; often one activity will be the inciting event that causes the tendon to swell. Rarely, multiple trigger fingers can be associated with rheumatoid arthritis in its early stages (see "Rheumatoid Arthritis," pages 89-90, for the details of the work-up).

RESULTS: These results were published by Anderson and Kaye (1991).

Table 5-1 Clinical Outcomes of 74 Cases of Trigger Finger Treated with D80, Followed Prospectively for 4.2 Years

Resolved with 1 injection	45 (61%)
Recurrence requiring 1 to 3 additional injections	20 (27%)
Failed to respond completely	9 (12%)
(Of the last 9 patients, surgical release was performed in 5 and 4 declined surgery)	
TOTAL	74

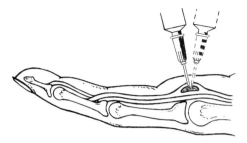

Enter directly over the palpable nodule
Needle: $^5/_8$-inch, 21- or 25-gauge
Depth: $^1/_4$ to $^3/_8$ inch into the cyst
Volume: 0.5 mL anesthetic
NOTE: After treatment apply manual
    pressure from either side to
    decompress the cyst

Figure 5-2A   Tendon cyst puncture and decompression.

SUMMARY
A tendon cyst is an abnormal collection of tenosynovial fluid either within the body of the tendon or adjacent to it. Direct, nonpenetrating trauma causes minor and reversible injury to the tendon or tendon sheath. This in turn leads to an overproduction of fluid that either collects inside the tendon or leaks out of the sheath with subsequent cyst formation. Despite its size (5 to 8 mm in diameter) and unlike its sister diagnosis trigger finger, the nodule rarely interferes with the function of the tendons or the adjacent joint. Flexion and extension of the finger are preserved.

TREATMENT OF CHOICE: Decompression is readily accomplished by simple puncture.

SEQUENCE OF TREATMENTS
1. Observation can be suggested; a significant number resolve without treatment.
2. *Acute restrictions:* Vibration exposure and direct pressure must be avoided (gloves or an adhesive pad placed over the cyst for protection).
3. *Injection:* Simple puncture with manual decompression is effective for all fluid-filled cysts (see details on page 78).
4. Cyst decompression can be repeated at 4 to 6 weeks and combined with injection of 0.25 mL triamcinolone acetonide 40 mg/mL (K40).
5. *Consultation:* Surgical consultation can be considered if the cyst has consistently interfered with the hand's function.

SURGICAL PROCEDURE: For cysts that remain symptomatic (pressure pain, interference with gripping and grasping, or persistent anxiety over its true nature), excision of the cyst can be considered. However, the patient must be advised of the possibility of postoperative tendon scarring that can lead to significant loss of range of motion of the tendon, the adjacent joint, or both.

INJECTION: Simple puncture and manual decompression is the treatment of choice for symptomatic cysts that do not resolve on their own.

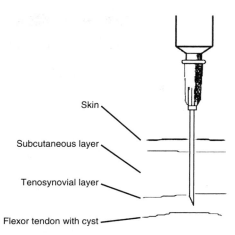

Skin

Subcutaneous layer

Tenosynovial layer

Flexor tendon with cyst

Figure 5-2B   Tendon cyst puncture.

Positioning: The hand is to be placed flat on the examination table with the palm up and the fingers outstretched.

Surface Anatomy and Point of Entry: The course of the flexor tendon is identified. The center of the tendon is marked both above and below the cyst. The cyst is palpated and marks are placed on either side of it. The point of entry is centered directly over the cyst.

Angle of Entry and Depth: The needle is inserted perpendicular to the skin. The depth of injection is $\frac{1}{4}$ to $\frac{3}{8}$ inch.

Anesthesia: Ethyl chloride is sprayed on the skin. Local anesthetic is placed in the subcutaneous tissue.

Technique: The cyst is identified by placing a fingertip above and a fingertip below. While holding the cyst firmly in place, the needle is centered over the nodule and passed down into the body of the cyst at least twice. The bevel of the needle is kept parallel to the tendon fibers (separating the tendon fibers rather than cutting them!). To ensure the accurate placement inside the cyst, the tendon can be passively flexed and extended; the needle should move with the cyst. Aspiration of the small amount of highly viscous fluid is usually unsuccessful. Manual pressure using the barrel of a syringe in a rolling fashion or with digital pressure will decompress most cysts. Less than 10% will not decompress with simple puncture (those that have very little fluid within the cyst cavity). The procedure can be repeated with a 21-gauge needle if the nodule size is not reduced.

INJECTION AFTERCARE

1. Movement of the finger *must be limited for the first 3 days* by avoiding all gripping, grasping, and direct pressure.
2. Immobilization of the adjacent two fingers with buddy-taping is an effective method of protecting the finger.
3. *Ice* (15 minutes every 4 to 6 hours), *acetaminophen* (1000 mg twice a day), or both, are used for postinjection soreness.
4. The finger must be *protected for 3 to 4 weeks* by avoiding repetitive gripping, grasping, pressure over the MCP heads, and vibration.

5. *Aspiration* can be repeated at 6 weeks and coupled with corticosteroid injection if the cyst fluid accumulates again.
6. Padded gloves or padded tools are suggested for long-term prevention in recurrent cases.
7. Observe (the cyst will often slowly undergo involution in size over several months).
8. Obtain a *consultation* with a surgical orthopedist if two consecutive punctures and time fail to resolve the condition; advise the patient of the possibility of postoperative scarring over the MCP joint that could adversely affect the range of motion of the finger!

OUTCOME AND FURTHER WORK-UP: Tenosynovial cysts are always the result of direct pressure or trauma over the flexor tendons as they course through the palm and down the finger. Work-up is not indicated. Radiographs are normal and the cysts are not an expression of any underlying systemic condition. Patients who develop recurrent cyst formation and those who develop multiple cysts, must attempt to identify the inciting activities or specific tasks that injure the flexor tendons.

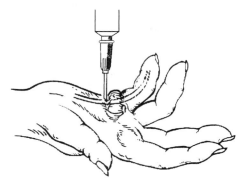

Enter adjacent to the nodular thickening in the midline over the flexor tendon; hold the needle vertically; injection is indicated only when tenosynovitis accompanies the fibrotic process
Needle: $^5/_8$-inch, 25-gauge
Depth: $^1/_2$ to $^3/_8$ inch
Volume: 0.5 mL anesthetic and 0.25 mL K40

Figure 5-3 Dupuytren's contracture injection.

SUMMARY

Dupuytren's contracture is a progressive fibrosis of the palmar fascia. Tissue thickening envelops the flexor tendons—typically the fourth and fifth tendons—and leads to a gradual flexion contracture of the fingers. The condition develops insidiously over decades. The initial tendon thickening often goes unnoticed and undiagnosed for years, gradually causing ever greater joint stiffness and palmar thickening. Many patients seek medical attention only after a significant degree of flexion contracture has occurred. The majority of cases are inherited, occurring more frequently in individuals of northern European descent. Chronic liver disease and postoperative scarring accounts for a small percentage of cases.

TREATMENT OF CHOICE: Although its efficacy has not been rigorously tested in the scientific literature, passive stretching of the flexor tendons after lanolin massage is the only treatment for patients with early palmar thickening. Tendon débridement and release is the treatment of choice when flexion contractures significantly interfere with hand function.

SEQUENCE OF TREATMENTS

1. *Exercise of choice:* Passive stretching of the flexor tendons after lanolin massage is used to maintain finger flexibility and range of motion.
2. Gloves or adhesive padding placed over the palmar thickening protects against irritation of direct pressure.
3. *Injection:* Corticosteroid injection with K40 is indicated only if tenosynovitis is present (see details on pages 75-76).
4. *Consultation:* Surgical consultation for débridement and tendon release can be considered if significant contracture has developed.

SURGICAL PROCEDURE: Significant finger contracture is treated with Z-plasty and partial fasciectomy (tendon débridement and release).

INJECTION: Less than 5% of cases have concomitant tenosynovitis. Local injection with corticosteroid is used only in these cases (see "Trigger Finger," pages 75-76).

OUTCOME AND FURTHER WORK-UP: Dupuytren's contracture is a slowly progressive condition. The scarring process continues despite stretching exercises and surgical débridement. Patients need to be advised of the relentless nature of the scarring and contracture process even after successful surgery. Although Dupuytren's contracture is associated with chronic liver disease and diabetes, 95% of cases are idiopathic with no underlying systemic disease. Further work-up is rarely indicated after diagnosing the condition; the scarring and contracture are typically a late manifestation of advanced cirrhosis of the liver and type 1 diabetes.

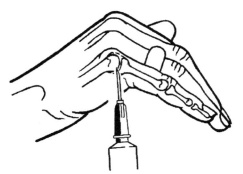

Enter over the joint line just distal to the metacarpal head, staying on the dorsal half of the joint
Needle: ⁵/₈-inch, 25-gauge
Depth: ¹/₄ to ³/₈ inch flush against the bone
Volume: 0.5 mL anesthetic and 0.25 mL K40
NOTE: The joint will not accept more than 0.25 mL; place the anesthetic in the subcutaneous tissue and the steroid just under the synovial membrane

Figure 5-4A   Arthrocentesis and injection of the metacarpophalangeal joint.

SUMMARY
Isolated arthritic involvement of the MCP joint is uncommon. The second and third MCP joints are affected most commonly. Swelling and inflammation of the joint are usually the result of remote and often unrecognized trauma—post-traumatic monarthric arthritis. Involvement of multiple MCP joints is more likely to be caused by rheumatoid arthritis. Septic arthritis of the MCP is rare; it is usually caused by penetrating injury. Aspiration of the joint is difficult and rarely produces enough fluid for analysis.

TREATMENT OF CHOICE: Joint swelling and inflammation respond much more favorably to corticosteroid injection than to nonsteroidal anti-inflammatory drugs (NSAIDs).

SEQUENCE OF TREATMENTS
1. Ice applied directly to the joint is effective for mild swelling.
2. *Acute restrictions:* Flexion and extension should be limited.
3. *Most common immobilizer:* A Velcro wrist immobilizer is convenient, but a radial gutter splint or an ulnar gutter splint provides better immobilization.
4. *Injection:* Corticosteroid injection with K40 is recommended for persistent nonseptic effusion (see details on page 83).
5. *Recovery exercises:* Passive stretching exercises in flexion and extension are performed for loss of range of motion and are followed by gripping exercises.

SURGICAL PROCEDURE: MCP implant arthroplasty (replacement) can be considered for joint involvement with severe loss of range of motion and strength.

INJECTION: Corticosteroid injection is the preferred anti-inflammatory treatment for nonseptic effusion. Note: The response to local corticosteroid injection depends on the extent of injury to the joint. If synovitis is accompanied by damage to the articular cartilage—pitted, fissured, or eroded cartilage (arthritic changes on radiographs)—injection will provide temporary benefit only.

Positioning: The hand is placed flat on the examination table with the palm down and the fingers outstretched.

Surface Anatomy and Point of Entry: The distal metacarpal head and the MCP joint line are identified either by palpating the joint line or alternatively subluxating the proximal phalangeal bone dorsally. The joint line is located $\frac{1}{4}$ inch beyond the prominence of the MCP knuckle! A 25-gauge needle is inserted into the skin over the distal metacarpal head adjacent to the joint line. For the second and fifth digits the point of entry will be just above the midplane, thus avoiding the neurovascular bundle. For the third and fourth digits the point of entry will be halfway between the MCP heads.

Angle of Entry and Depth: The needle is inserted perpendicular to the skin for the second and fifth digits and at a 45-degree angle for the third and fourth digits. The depth of injection is $\frac{1}{4}$ to $\frac{3}{8}$ inch.

Anesthesia: Ethyl chloride is sprayed on the skin. Local anesthetic is placed in the subcutaneous tissue (0.5 mL).

Technique: A **dorsal approach** is preferable. The needle is advanced until the firm resistance of the supporting ligament and the joint capsule is encountered. Anesthesia is injected just outside this layer ($\frac{1}{8}$ inch). Then the needle is advanced to the hard resistance of the bone ($\frac{1}{4}$ inch) and 0.25 mL of K40 is injected under the synovial membrane. Note: These small joints can accommodate only a small volume of medication. If the pressure of injection increases, withdraw $\frac{1}{16}$ inch.

INJECTION AFTERCARE
1. The joint must be ***protected for the first 3 days*** by avoiding direct pressure and all gripping, grasping, extremes of motion, vibration, and cold.
2. ***Ice*** (15 minutes every 4 to 6 hours), ***acetaminophen*** (1000 mg twice a day), or both, are used for postinjection soreness.

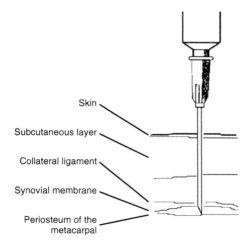

Skin
Subcutaneous layer
Collateral ligament
Synovial membrane
Periosteum of the metacarpal

Figure 5-4B Injection of the metacarpophalangeal joint.

3. The motion of the fingers must be *limited for 3 to 4 weeks* by avoiding repetitive gripping, grasping, pressure over the MCP heads, and vibration or alternatively with a Velcro wrist immobilizer with metal stay for advanced disease.
4. Begin passive *stretching exercises* in flexion and extension at 2 to 3 weeks.
5. Begin isometric *gripping exercises* at 4 to 5 weeks.
6. The *injection* can be repeated at 6 weeks with corticosteroid if swelling persists or range of motion is still limited.
7. Padded gloves or padded tools are strongly suggested for long-term prevention in recurrent cases.
8. A *consultation* with a surgical orthopedist can be considered if two consecutive injections fail to improve the condition and range of motion remains impaired.

OUTCOME AND FURTHER WORK-UP: Isolated involvement of one or two MCP joints is uniformly caused by trauma. Although close inspection and width measurement of the articular cartilage on plain film radiographs of the hands is the best way to determine the severity and prognosis of the condition, ultimately the long-term outcome will depend on how effective treatment controls the inflammatory response and the ability of the body to smooth over any damaged cartilage. Symmetric involvement of the MCPs of both hands is the classic presentation of an inflammatory arthritis. These patients require a complete joint examination and laboratory testing to define the specific rheumatic condition.

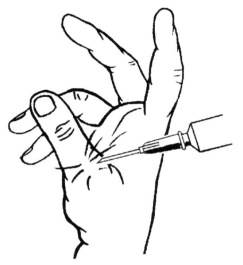

Enter $^1/_4$ inch distal to the prominence
of the distal metacarpal head on the
ulnar side of the joint; use
anesthesia to differentiate this
ligament injury from acute arthritis
Needle: $^5/_8$-inch, 25-gauge
Depth: between $^1/_8$ and $^1/_4$ inch, just
under the skin and above the ulnar
collateral ligament
Volume: 0.25 mL of anesthetic
(corticosteroid is not used for this
condition)
NOTE: In order to locate the proper
depth of injection, advance the
needle to the hard resistance of the
bone and then withdraw $^1/_8$ inch

Figure 5-5A   Gamekeeper's thumb—ulnar collateral ligament injury of the metacarpal joint.

SUMMARY

The gamekeeper of the royal court was likely to injure the ulnar collateral ligament of the
metacarpophalangeal (MP) joint when twisting the necks of the fowl hunted for the king. Today,
ski pole injuries are the most common cause of this condition. Whether by injury or repetitive use,
the disrupted ligament leads to instability of the MP joint, poor pinching and opposition function
of the thumb, and in later years degenerative arthritis.

TREATMENT OF CHOICE: Immobilization with a dorsal hood splint or thumb spica cast is
the treatment of choice for this ligament injury.

SEQUENCE OF TREATMENTS

1. Ice is applied in the first few days to reduce the swelling at the MP joint.
2. *Acute restrictions:* Restriction of pinching, gripping, and grasping is begun immediately.
3. *Most common immobilizers:* A dorsal hood splint or thumb spica cast is worn for 4 to 6 weeks
   to allow reattachment of the ligament.
4. *Injection:* Local anesthetic block is used to confirm the diagnosis; corticosteroid is not used for
   this injury.
5. *Recovery exercises:* Gentle stretching exercises of the thumb to restore flexion and extension
   are begun after the cast is removed.
6. *Consultation:* Consultation with an orthopedic hand specialist is recommended if the thumb
   remains unstable and with poor function.

SURGICAL PROCEDURE: Either reattachment of the torn distal ligament, tendon graft repair, or fusion of the joint (arthrodesis) is performed depending on the severity of the injury and the length symptoms have been present.

OUTCOME AND FURTHER WORK-UP: The outcome of this injury depends on the severity of the ligament injury and whether injury to the underlying articular cartilage has occurred concomitantly. Those patients who exhibit persistent swelling and impaired motion of the joint despite signs of ligament healing have likely injured articular cartilage. These patients have the greatest risk of future arthritic deterioration.

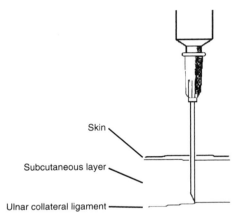

Skin

Subcutaneous layer

Ulnar collateral ligament

Figure 5-5B Gamekeeper's thumb injection.

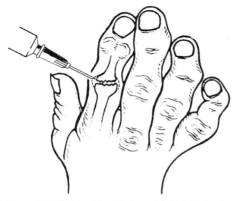

The proximal interphalangeal (PIP)
joint accepts medication much more
readily than the distal
interphalangeal (DIP) joint; enter at
the joint line, $\frac{1}{4}$ inch beyond the
distal end of the proximal phalanges
above the midplane
Needle: $\frac{5}{8}$-inch, 25-gauge
Depth: $\frac{1}{4}$ to $\frac{3}{8}$ inch, flush against the
adjacent bone
Volume: 0.25 to 0.5 mL anesthetic and
0.125 mL K40
NOTE: Use small amounts of
anesthetic in the superficial layers;
the joint will accept only small
volumes

Figure 5-6   Proximal interphalangeal joint injection in osteoarthritis of the hand.

SUMMARY

Osteoarthritis of the small joints of the hands is a universal problem. It is characterized by relatively painless bony enlargement and deformity at the DIP joints (Heberden's nodes) and of the PIP joints (Bouchard's nodes). Radiographs demonstrate a variable degree of asymmetric wear of the articular cartilage, bony osteophytes along the margins of the joint line, and subchondral sclerosis. A family history, heavy use, and repeated exposure to vibration are all associated with an increased susceptibility.

SEQUENCE OF TREATMENTS

1. *Acute restrictions:* Restriction of the extremes of position, cold exposure, and vibration exposure will reduce the achiness and irritation of the affected joints.
2. The intensity of pinching, gripping, and grasping should be limited.
3. Oral extra-strength acetaminophen (1 g twice a day) or oral enteric-coated aspirin (8 to 12 325-mg enteric-coated aspirins per day in divided doses) are the safest long-term medications; use of the NSAIDs is reserved for acute flare-ups.
4. Capsaicin cream or a moderate concentrated cortisone cream is massaged directly over the joint.
5. *Exercise of choice:* Gentle range of motion exercises using manual movement or Chinese chime balls is a practical method of maintaining function.
6. *Injection:* Injection with K40 can provide temporary relief of an acutely swollen joint (see details on page 90).

INJECTION: Occasionally an isolated small joint of the hand will present with enlargement, pain, and swelling that is disproportionate to the other joints of the hand (enough swelling to interfere with the full flexion of the joint). A history of trauma is often obtained. The symptoms gradually develop over weeks, as opposed to the acute presentation of a monarthric septic arthritis occurring over hours or days. This monarthric traumatic arthritis is an acute flare of an underlying osteoarthritic joint and is often very responsive to intra-articular injection.

OUTCOME AND FURTHER WORK-UP: Arthritis affecting a single joint is nearly always a result of previous trauma. The associated swelling and loss of range of motion usually respond well to a combination of injection and immobilization, but only temporarily. Recurrent arthritic flares are the rule depending on the patient's occupation, extracurricular activities, and arthritic wear-and-tear on radiograph. Arthritis involving multiple joints deserves a laboratory work-up for rheumatoid, psoriatic, or lupus-based arthritis.

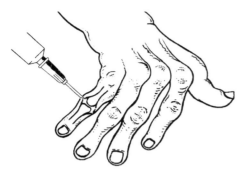

Enter at the joint line above the
  midplane
Needle: $\frac{5}{8}$-inch, 25-gauge
Depth: $\frac{1}{4}$ to $\frac{3}{8}$ inch
Volume: 0.25 to 0.5 mL anesthetic in
  the subcutaneous tissues and 0.125
  to 0.25 mL K40 flush against the
  bone
NOTE: Do not insert the needle
  between the articular surfaces of the
  joint (damaging); with the needle
  held gently against the bone, the
  medication will be injected under
  the synovial membrane and hence
  will be intra-articular

Figure 5-7A   Proximal interphalangeal joint injection in rheumatoid arthritis.

SUMMARY

Rheumatoid arthritis (RA) is an inflammatory arthritis that has several unique presentations. Classic RA is characterized by a symmetric, polyarticular, small-joint arthritis affecting the MCP, PIP, and metatarsophalangeal (MTP) joints. The affected joints demonstrate moderately intense inflammation, fusiform swelling, and synovial thickening. Non-classic RA can affect just a single joint (monarthric), several medium-size to large joints (pauciarticular), or several small joints that remain inflamed and swollen for just a few days (palindromic). Systemic treatment with oral medications—aspirin, NSAIDs, methotrexate, hydroxychloroquine sulfate (Plaquenil Sulfate), oral corticosteroids—remains the mainstay of treatment.

TREATMENT OF CHOICE: Systemic treatment with oral medication.

SEQUENCE OF TREATMENTS
1. Ice applied directly to the joint(s) can reduce pain and swelling.
2. *Acute restrictions:* The affected joints must be restricted in flexion and extension.
3. Appropriate immobilization is applied to the most involved joints (buddy-taping the PIP joints); radial or ulnar gutter splint (MCP joints); or Velcro wrist immobilizer with metal stay.
4. *Injection:* Aspiration is used for diagnosis; corticosteroid injection with K40 is an appropriate initial treatment for localized disease affecting one or two joints.
5. *Exercise of choice:* Once the inflammation is controlled, passive range of motion exercises are performed.
6. *Consultation:* Surgical consultation is reserved for advanced disease with functional loss due to deformity.

SURGICAL PROCEDURE: Implant arthroplasty of the PIP joints (replacement) is performed for severe deformity associated with a loss of function.

INJECTION: Many patients with early presentations of rheumatoid arthritis, especially the monarthric and pauciarticular forms, can be successfully managed with local corticosteroid injection.

89

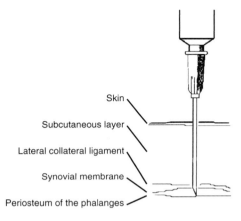

Skin

Subcutaneous layer

Lateral collateral ligament

Synovial membrane

Periosteum of the phalanges

Figure 5-7B Proximal interphalangeal joint injection.

Positioning: The hand is placed flat with the palm down and the fingers extended.

Surface Anatomy and Point of Entry: The head of the proximal phalanges is located and marked. The joint line of the PIP joint is $\frac{1}{4}$ inch distal to the most prominent portion of the head of the proximal phalanges. The point of entry is adjacent to the joint line.

Angle of Entry and Depth: The needle is inserted perpendicular to the skin. The depth of injection is $\frac{1}{4}$ to $\frac{3}{8}$ inch.

Anesthesia: Ethyl chloride is sprayed on the skin. Because the depth of the synovial membrane is so superficial, injection of local anesthetic in the subcutaneous tissue (0.25 mL) is optional. The tissues sounding the small joints of the hand can only accommodate a small volume, so anesthesia should be kept to a minimum.

Technique: This technique uses an **indirect method** of injecting cortisone into the joint, taking advantage of the anatomic attachment of the synovial membrane to the adjacent bone. The synovial membrane is approximately 1 cm long (see Fig. 5-7A). Instead of attempting to inject into the center of the joint, which is difficult, painful, and potentially dangerous (cartilage damage), the 25-gauge needle is advanced through the synovial membrane and down to the bone adjacent to the joint line. The center of the joint is *not* entered directly. With the needle held flush against the bone, the medication is injected under the synovial membrane. Moderate pressure may be needed. If high pressure is required, especially if the patient experiences pain with injection, the needle is withdrawn $\frac{1}{16}$ inch.

INJECTION AFTERCARE

1. The joint must be *protected for the first 3 days* by avoiding direct pressure and all gripping, grasping, extremes of motion, vibration, and cold.
2. Buddy-taping to the adjacent PIP joint or a finger splint can be used for the first few days.
3. *Ice* (15 minutes every 4 to 6 hours), *acetaminophen* (1000 mg twice a day), or both, are used for postinjection soreness.
4. The motion of the fingers must be *limited for 3 to 4 weeks* by avoiding repetitive gripping, grasping, and pinching.

5. Passive range of motion ***stretching exercises*** in flexion and extension are begun at 2 to 3 weeks.
6. ***Gripping exercises*** are performed at 4 to 5 weeks.
7. The ***injection*** can be repeated at 6 weeks if swelling persists or range of motion is still affected.
8. Padded gloves or padded tools are suggested for long-term prevention in recurrent cases.

OUTCOME AND FURTHER WORK-UP: Many patients with early presentations of rheumatoid arthritis, especially the monarthric and pauciarticular forms, can be successfully managed with local corticosteroid injection. However, if the disease progresses to multiple joint involvement, systemic treatment with oral medication should be initiated. The decision to start hydroxychloroquine sulfate, gold, penicillamine, or methotrexate should not be delayed. These remitting drugs may take months to have an appreciable clinical effect.

Chapter 6

CHEST

THE DIFFERENTIAL DIAGNOSIS OF CHEST PAIN

DIAGNOSES	CONFIRMATIONS
Rib cage (most common)	
Costochondritis	Local anesthetic block
Sternochondritis	Local anesthetic block
Tietze's syndrome	Examination
Endemic pleurodynia	Examination; local anesthetic block
Rib fracture, nondisplaced	Chest compression sign, chest radiograph, or bone scan
Rib fracture, displaced	Chest compression sign, chest radiograph
Sternum	
Sternoclavicular joint strain	Local anesthetic block
Inflammatory arthritis	Local anesthetic block; abnormal erythrocyte sedimentation rate; examination correlations
Septic (intravenous drug use)	Aspiration and culture
Referred pain to the chest wall	
Hiatal hernia	Gastrointestinal cocktail taken orally; barium swallow; endoscopy
Cholelithiasis	Liver chemistries; ultrasound
Splenic flexure syndrome	Examination; radiograph of abdomen
Coronary artery disease	Electrocardiogram; creatine phosphokinase, troponin, or angiogram
Aortic aneurysm	Computed tomography (CT) scan of the chest; angiogram
Pneumonia	Chest radiograph; complete blood count, cultures
Pulmonary embolism	Oxygen saturation; D-dimer, lung scan; CT scan or angiogram

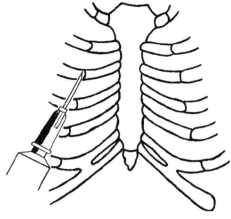

Enter atop the center of the rib; angle
the syringe perpendicular to the skin
Needle: $\frac{5}{8}$-inch, 25-gauge
Depth: $\frac{1}{2}$ to 1 inch, depending on the
location on the chest
Volume: 1 to 2 mL of local anesthetic
and 0.5 mL of either D80 or K40
NOTE: The injections should be placed
flush against the cartilage adjacent
to the costochondral junction using
mild pressure

Figure 6-1A   Injection of the costochondral cartilage.

SUMMARY

Inflammation of the cartilage of the chest wall can occur either at the junction of the rib and the costal cartilage, *costochondritis*, or at the junction of the costal cartilage and the sternum, *sternochondritis*. Local tenderness of the chest wall and pain with chest compression are the hallmark findings on examination. The diagnosis can be confirmed with local anesthetic block placed at the junction of the cartilage and bone. Most cases resolve slowly over 4 to 6 weeks. Corticosteroid injection is occasionally necessary for the uncommon case that persists.

TREATMENT OF CHOICE: Because most cases resolve spontaneously, the treatment of choice is simple observation. Corticosteroid injection is the preferred treatment for symptoms that have been present for more than 4 to 6 weeks.

SEQUENCE OF TREATMENTS

1. A period of observation for several weeks is warranted because many cases will resolve without treatment.
2. Patients with this condition always need reassurance, that it is not a heart condition.
3. *Acute restrictions:* Chest expansion, coughing, reaching, lifting, pushing, and pulling must be restricted.
4. *Most common immobilizer:* A chest binder or a wide, well-fitted bra is an effective immobilizer.
5. *Injection:* Diagnostic anesthetic injection is used to confirm the diagnosis (hence making the diagnosis of coronary artery disease less likely) combined with corticosteroid injection with depot methylprednisolone 80 mg/mL (D80) if symptoms have failed to resolve in 6 to 8 weeks (see details on page 94).

SURGICAL PROCEDURE: None.

INJECTION: Local anesthetic injection is used to differentiate the pain arising from the chest wall from coronary artery pain, pleurisy, or other causes of chest pain. Corticosteroid injection is used to treat symptoms that persist beyond 6 to 8 weeks.

Positioning: The patient is placed in the supine position.

Surface Anatomy and the Point of Entry: The point of maximum chest wall tenderness is carefully palpated. The center point of the cartilage is identified by placing one finger above and one finger below the cartilage in the intercostal spaces. The point of entry for sternochondritis is 1 inch from the midline of the sternum, directly over the center of the rib. The point of entry for costochondritis is over the point of maximum tenderness along the course of the rib.

Angle of Entry and Depth: The needle is inserted perpendicular to the skin. The depth of injection is $\frac{1}{2}$ inch for sternochondritis and $\frac{1}{2}$ to 1 inch for costochondritis.

Anesthesia: Ethyl chloride is sprayed on the skin. Local anesthetic is placed in the subcutaneous tissue (0.5 mL) and just above the firm resistance of the cartilage or hard resistance of the bone.

Technique: Successful treatment depends on the identification of the most involved costal cartilage and the accurate localization of the junction of the cartilage and the bone. The most affected costal cartilage is identified either by careful palpation of the most painful junction or by local anesthetic block. After anesthesia, an **indirect method** of injection is used to place the corticosteroid. This method takes advantage of the anatomic attachment of the synovial membrane attached to the rib and costal cartilage. The synovial membrane is approximately 1 cm long. Instead of attempting to advance into the center of the joint, which is difficult, painful, and potentially damaging, the 25-gauge needle is advanced through the synovial membrane and down either to the hard resistance of the bone or the firm resistance of the cartilage adjacent to the joint line. The center of the joint is *not* entered directly. With the needle held flush against the bone or cartilage, 0.5 mL of triamcinolone acetonide 40 mg/mL (K40) or D80 is injected under the synovial membrane.

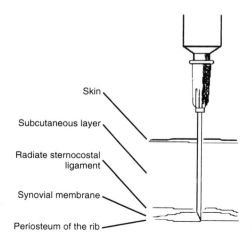

Skin

Subcutaneous layer

Radiate sternocostal
ligament

Synovial membrane

Periosteum of the rib

Figure 6-1B Costochondritis injection.

94

INJECTION AFTERCARE

1. The chest wall must be *protected for the first 3 days* by avoiding direct pressure, lying on the sides, lifting, and strenuous activities.
2. The injection is combined with a rib binder (or wide bra) for the first few days (especially for persistent or recurrent cases).
3. *Ice* (15 minutes every 4 to 6 hours), *acetaminophen (Tylenol ES)* (1000 mg twice a day), or both, are used for postinjection soreness.
4. The chest wall must be *protected* for 3 to 4 weeks by limiting lying on the sides, lifting, and strenuous activities, and aggressively treating coughing and sneezing.
5. The *injection* can be repeated at 6 weeks if local irritation continues.

OUTCOME AND FURTHER WORK-UP: Because most cases resolve spontaneously within 4 to 6 weeks, specific treatments may not be necessary. Few cases will require corticosteroid injection. Work-up is unnecessary in most cases. If symptoms are only partially controlled with local anesthesia, continued search for a second cause of chest pain is warranted.

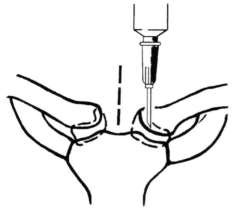

Enter atop the center of the proximal
   clavicle with the needle
   perpendicular to the skin
Needle: $\frac{5}{8}$-inch, 25-gauge
Depth: $\frac{3}{8}$ to $\frac{1}{2}$ inch
Volume: 1 mL of local anesthetic and
   0.5 mL K40
NOTE: The injection should be placed
   flush against the proximal end of the
   clavicle, just adjacent to the center
   of the joint using mild pressure

Figure 6-2A   Sternoclavicular joint injection.

SUMMARY

Anterior swelling and inflammation of the sternoclavicular (SC) joint is uncommon. Mild to moderate swelling of the joint and pseudoenlargement of the proximal end of the clavicle occur most commonly as a consequence of either acute or remote trauma. Moderate inflammatory change can occur in Reiter's disease. Septic arthritis with severe swelling, redness, and pain is an unusual complication of intravenous drug abuse.

TREATMENT OF CHOICE: Ice applications combined with restrictions of shoulder adduction and sleeping on the affected side are the treatments of choice.

SEQUENCE OF TREATMENTS

1. Ice is placed directly over the joint.
2. *Acute restrictions:* Shoulder adduction, reaching, and the direct pressure of sleeping on the affected side are restricted.
3. *Most common immobilizer:* A shoulder immobilizer can be used for 3 to 4 weeks.
4. *Injection:* Injection with local anesthetic can be used alone to confirm the diagnosis or combined with corticosteroid injection (K40) for symptoms that have persisted for more than 6 to 8 weeks (see details on page 97).
5. *Recovery exercise:* General shoulder conditioning excluding exercises that involve reaching at or above the shoulder is indicated when the acute symptoms have resolved.

SURGICAL PROCEDURE: None.

INJECTION: Local anesthetic injection is used to identify the sternoclavicular joint as the source of anterior chest wall swelling or pain. This is especially necessary when the patient complains that *"the bone is growing"*—the pseudoenlargement of the proximal clavicle. Corticosteroid injection is used to treat symptoms that have persisted beyond 6 to 8 weeks.

Positioning: The patient is to be in the supine position.

Surface Anatomy and the Point of Entry: The midline, the sternal notch, and the center of the proximal clavicle are identified and marked. The point of entry is $^3/_4$ to 1 inch from the midline, directly over the center of the proximal clavicle.

Angle of Entry and Depth: The needle is inserted perpendicular to the skin. The depth of injection is $^3/_8$ to $^1/_2$ inch.

Anesthesia: Ethyl chloride is sprayed on the skin. Local anesthetic is placed in the subcutaneous tissue (0.25 mL) and just above the firm to hard resistance of the periosteum of the bone (0.25 mL).

Technique: The success of treatment depends on the accurate localization of the point of entry. After confirming the diagnosis with local anesthesia, the syringe containing the anesthetic is replaced with the second syringe containing 0.5 mL of K40. The needle is advanced down to the hard resistance of the clavicle. With just the weight of the syringe against the periosteum, the corticosteroid is injected flush against the bone. This is another example of the **indirect method** of injection of a small joint. Taking advantage of the 1-cm-long synovial membrane that attaches to the adjacent clavicle and bone, the 25-gauge needle is held flush against the clavicle and the medication is injected under the synovial membrane and hence into the joint.

INJECTION AFTERCARE
1. The joint must be ***protected for the first 3 days*** by avoiding sleeping on the affected side, reaching, lifting, and all strenuous activities.
2. ***Ice*** (15 minutes every 4 to 6 hours), ***acetaminophen*** (1000 mg twice a day), or both, are used for postinjection soreness.

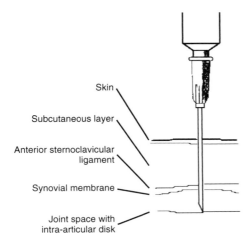

Skin

Subcutaneous layer

Anterior sternoclavicular ligament

Synovial membrane

Joint space with intra-articular disk

Figure 6-2B   Sternoclavicular joint injection.

97

3. Movement of the joint must be *limited* for 3 to 4 weeks by restricting sleeping on the affected side, reaching, lifting, and all strenuous activities.
4. The injection can be combined with a shoulder immobilizer for 3 to 7 days for persistent or recurrent cases.
5. The *injection* can be repeated at 6 weeks if swelling persists or range of motion remains impaired.

OUTCOME AND FURTHER WORK-UP: Most patients who present with a swollen SC joint are disturbed by the appearance of an enlarging bone. Apical lordotic views of the clavicles will confirm the normal size of the bones. Local anesthetic block is an integral part of the diagnosis and is very helpful in allaying the patient's anxiety over the condition (the bone appears larger because of the deep swelling that forces the bone outward).

THE DIFFERENTIAL DIAGNOSIS OF LOWER BACK PAIN

DIAGNOSES	CONFIRMATIONS
Lumbosacral back strain (most common)	
Unaccustomed or improper use	Examination: local tenderness; Schöber's measurement
Reactive lumbosacral back strain	
Osteoarthritis	Radiographs: routine back series
Scoliosis	Radiographs: standing scoliosis views
Spondylolisthesis	Radiographs: routine back series and the oblique views
Herniated disk	Computed tomography (CT) scanning or magnetic resonance imaging (MRI)
Compression fracture	Radiographs: lateral view of the back; bone scan; MRI
Epidural process	MRI
Lumbosacral radiculopathy ("sciatica")	
Herniated disk	CT scanning or MRI
Osteoarthritis-spinal stenosis	CT scanning or MRI
Intra-abdominal process	Ultrasound or CT scanning
Wallet sciatica	History
Sacroiliac joint	
Strain	Local anesthetic block
Sacroiliitis	Radiographs: standing anteroposterior pelvis; oblique views of the sacroiliac joints; bone scan
Referred pain	
Kidney (pyelonephritis, stones, etc.)	Urinalysis; intravenous pyelogram; ultrasound, etc.
Aorta	Ultrasound
Colon (appendicitis, cecal carcinoma, rectal carcinoma, etc.)	Hemoccult; barium enema; etc.
Pelvis (tumor, pregnancy, etc.)	Examination; ultrasound; etc.

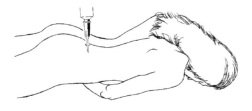

Occasionally a patient presents with very localized tenderness in the erector spinae muscle; dramatic relief with local anesthesia is the best indication for corticosteroid injection
Needle: 1½-inch, 22-gauge
Depth: 1¼ to 1½ inches
Volume: 2 to 3 mL anesthetic and 1 mL D80
NOTE: Place the anesthesia at the first tissue plane—the erector spinae fascia—then enter the muscle three times to cover an area of approximately 1 inch horizontally

Figure 7-1A Acute lumbosacral back muscle injection.

SUMMARY

Lumbosacral strain is a spasm and irritation of the supporting muscles of the lumbar spine. Although lumbosacral strain can occur as an isolated problem of overuse of improperly stretched and toned muscles, a significant proportion has an underlying cause, such as scoliosis, spondylolisthesis, osteoarthritis, compression fracture, or radiculopathy.

TREATMENT OF CHOICE: Bed rest, physical therapy exercises, and a muscle relaxer are used as the initial treatment.

SEQUENCE OF TREATMENTS

1. Ice is applied to the lower back muscles.
2. *Acute restrictions:* The acute phase of treatment combines 3 to 4 days of bed rest, no greater than 30 minutes of walking or standing when out of bed, and restriction of bending, twisting, and lifting.
3. An oral muscle relaxer in a dosage sufficient to cause mild sedation is recommended but used only when the patient is recumbent.
4. Pain medication is prescribed for the first 7 to 10 days.
5. *Exercises of choice:* The lower back is heated and the flexion stretching exercises are performed daily (knee-chest pulls, side bends, and pelvic rocks).
6. Crutches or a walker is strongly advised after the obligate period of bed rest.
7. *Most common immobilizer:* A Velcro lumbosacral corset is used to support the spine.
8. *Injection:* Local corticosteroid injection with depot methylprednisolone 80 mg/mL (D80) is recommended for persistent focal muscle irritation.
9. *Recovery exercises:* Flexion stretching exercises are combined with muscle toning exercises (modified sit-ups and weighted side bends) and general light aerobic exercise to complete the recovery.

SURGICAL PROCEDURE: Surgery is considered only when an underlying, correctable cause is identified, such as subtle disk, spondylolisthesis, scoliosis, and so forth.

INJECTION: Local injection of the paraspinal muscles or the lumbar facet joints is infrequently used and of questionable overall value. Occasionally a patient will present with very localized tenderness in the erector spinae and respond to local anesthesia. Dramatic relief with anesthesia is the best indication for corticosteroid injection.

Positioning: The patient is placed in the prone position, completely flat.

Surface Anatomy and the Point of Entry: The spinous processes of the lumbosacral spine are marked. The point of entry is $1\frac{1}{2}$ inches from the midline, directly over the point of maximum muscle tenderness at the convexity of the paraspinous muscle.

Angle of Entry and Depth: The needle is inserted perpendicular to the skin. The depth of injection is $1\frac{1}{4}$ to $1\frac{1}{2}$ inches.

Anesthesia: Ethyl chloride is sprayed on the skin. Local anesthetic is placed in the subcutaneous tissue (0.5 mL), just above the moderate resistance of the outer fascia of the muscle (1 mL) and in the muscle belly itself (1 to 2 mL).

Technique: The success of treatment depends of the accurate injection of the affected muscle. A 22-gauge, $1\frac{1}{2}$-inch needle is passed vertically down to the firm rubbery resistance of the outer fascia of the muscle, approximately 1 to $1\frac{1}{4}$ inches deep. The muscle is entered three times in an area the size of a quarter. A total of 2 or 3 mL of local anesthetic is injected. The needle is withdrawn and local tenderness, range of motion, or both are reevaluated. If pain and function are improved, the muscle can be injected with 1 mL of D80. However, local anesthetic injection, either to confirm the diagnosis or to treat the acute case of lumbosacral strain, can be used alone.

INJECTION AFTERCARE

1. The back must be *protected for the first 3 days* by avoiding direct pressure, bending, twisting, and all unnecessary walking and standing.

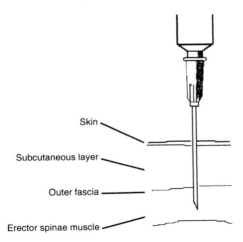

Skin

Subcutaneous layer

Outer fascia

Erector spinae muscle

Figure 7-1B   Erector spinae muscle injection.

101

2. Three days of bed rest with the use of crutches with touch-down weightbearing is strongly recommended for severe cases.
3. *Ice* (15 minutes every 4 to 6 hours), *acetaminophen (Tylenol ES)* (1000 mg twice a day), or both, are used for postinjection soreness.
4. Movement of the back must be *limited* for 3 to 4 weeks by restricting repetitive bending, lifting, twisting, and all unnecessary walking and standing.
5. A lumbosacral corset is prescribed for the first 2 to 3 weeks for recurrent or severe cases.
6. Passive *stretching exercises* in flexion are begun when the acute pain has begun to resolve (knee-chest pulls, pelvic rocks, and side bends).
7. The *injection* can be repeated at 6 weeks with corticosteroid if pain and muscle spasm persist.
8. Active *toning exercises* of the abdominal and lower back muscle are begun only once flexibility has been restored.
9. *Plain film radiographs* or *CT/MRI* is obtained to identify the subtle disk, progressive spondylolisthesis, acquired scoliosis, or other correctable conditions in the patient with chronic symptoms.

OUTCOME AND FURTHER WORK-UP: Most episodes of lumbosacral strain resolve completely with a combination of rest, stretching exercises, a muscle relaxer, and injection. However, because the muscle spasm of the supporting muscle of the spine can be a reaction to an underlying threat to the spinal column, cord, or nerve, any patient with recurrent or severe strain must be evaluated for underlying structural back disease, lumbar radiculopathy, spinal stenosis, and so forth. Plain films of the lumbar spine, CT scanning, MRI, or electromyography (EMG) testing complete the work-up.

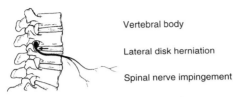

Vertebral body

Lateral disk herniation

Spinal nerve impingement

Figure 7-2   Herniated disk of the lumbar spine.

SUMMARY
Sciatica is the term commonly used to describe the pain associated with the compression of the lumbosacral nerve roots or of one of the nerves of the lumbosacral plexus. Pressure on the nerve from a herniated disk, from bony osteophytes (spinal stenosis with narrowing of the lateral recess), a compression fracture, or any other extrinsic pressure (for example, epidural process, pelvic mass, or wallet sciatica) causes progressive sensory, sensorimotor, or sensorimotor visceral symptoms. Minor degrees of nerve compression—sensory only sciatica—is more likely to improve with conservative management (see "Lumbosacral Strain," page 100). Sensorimotor sciatica requires early radiographic study, more aggressive treatment, and depending on the degree and progressive of neurologic function, surgical intervention. However, sciatica-associated motor or bowel and bladder symptoms—the most severe degree of neurologic dysfunction—is an emergent problem that requires immediate study, surgical consultation, and often surgical treatment. Selected cases of chronic sensory sciatica respond to an epidural injection of an anesthetic and corticosteroid. This procedure should be performed by an anesthesiologist or interventional radiologist.

TREATMENT OF CHOICE: Bed rest, physical therapy exercises, and a muscle relaxer can be used as the initial treatments in mild to moderate cases of sciatica (patients with high-grade neurologic dysfunction should undergo radiographic study and early surgical consultation).

SEQUENCE OF TREATMENTS
1. Ice placed over the lower back muscles is an effective analgesic and muscle relaxant.
2. *Acute restrictions:* Three to 4 days of bed rest, including a daily limitation of 30 minutes of walking and standing, is combined with restrictions of bending, twisting, and lifting.
3. An oral muscle relaxer in a dosage sufficient to cause mild sedation is recommended but used only when the patient is recumbent.
4. Adequate pain medication is prescribed for 7 to 10 days.
5. *Injection:* Local corticosteroid injection with D80 can be used for persistent focal muscle irritation, or the selected nerve root can be treated with an epidural injection of D80.
6. *Exercises of choice:* Passive stretching exercises of the lower back in flexion are performed after heat applications (knee-chest pulls, side bends, and pelvic rocks) and combined with McKensie extension exercises as tolerated.
7. The use of crutches or a walker is strongly recommended as a transition to greater weightbearing after the obligate period of bed rest.
8. *Most common immobilizer:* A Velcro lumbosacral corset is used during the transitional period

or for the recurrent or chronic case.

9. ***Recovery exercises:*** Passive stretching exercises in flexion are combined with muscle toning exercises (modified sit-ups and weighted side bends) and general light aerobic exercise to complete the recovery.

SURGICAL PROCEDURE: In the setting of persistent or progressive neurologic dysfunction (especially involving loss of bowel or bladder control and motor weakness), diskectomy (herniated disk), decompression laminectomy (for spinal stenosis), and surgical fusion (unstable compression fracture) are the most common procedures.

INJECTION: Local injection of the paraspinal muscles or the lumbar facet joints is infrequently used and of questionable overall value. Occasionally a patient will present with very localized tenderness in the erector spinae and respond dramatically to local anesthesia and corticosteroid injection (see page 101).

OUTCOME AND FURTHER WORK-UP: The history and neurologic examination are used to stage lumbar radiculopathy. Imaging studies are used to define the anatomy and distinguish herniated nucleus pulposus (HNP) from spinal stenosis, spondylolisthesis, and epidural abscess. EMG is used to further define the extent of neurologic impairment and distinguish involvement of one spinal level from another. The outcome of lumbar radiculopathy depends on the degree of neurologic impairment on examination, the length of time the nerve has been under pressure, the underlying process (HNP, spinal stenosis, epidural abscess, etc.), and the age and general medical condition of the patient.

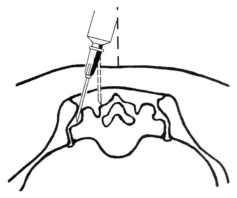

Enter 1 inch caudal to the posterior
superior iliac spine (PSIS) and
1 inch lateral to the midline;
advance at a 70-degree angle to
the firm resistance of the posterior
supporting ligaments
Needle: $1\frac{1}{2}$-inch or $3\frac{1}{2}$-inch,
22-gauge
Depth: $1\frac{1}{2}$ to $2\frac{1}{2}$ inches
Volume: 1 to 2 mL local anesthetic
and 1 mL K40
NOTE: The injection should be placed
flush against the periosteum at the
junction of the sacrum and the
ileum at the maximum depth

Figure 7-3A   Sacroiliac joint injection.

SUMMARY

Sacroiliac strain is an injury and sacroiliitis is a rheumatic inflammation of the articulation between the sacrum and the ileum. Sacroiliac strain results from the mechanical irritation of improper lifting, twisting injuries, seat belt injury, or direct trauma. Sacroiliitis is most often associated with the spondyloarthropathies including, Reiter's disease, ankylosing spondylitis, and ulcerative colitis–associated arthritis. Septic arthritis of the sacroiliac joint is rare. Regardless of cause, symptoms of this unique cause of low back pain are generally very well localized to the lower back. Less commonly, symptoms can be referred into the gluteal area or down the back of the leg, mimicking sciatica.

TREATMENT OF CHOICE: Rest is combined with physical therapy exercises.

SEQUENCE OF TREATMENTS

1. Ice placed over the lower sacrum is often tried but is only partially effective because of the depth of the joint.
2. *Acute restrictions:* Three to 4 days of bed rest is combined with 2 to 4 weeks of restricted bending, twisting, and lifting.
3. An oral muscle relaxer is prescribed while at bed rest; the dosage must be sufficient to cause mild sedation.
4. Pain medication is used for 7 to 10 days.
5. *Exercises of choice:* The lower back is heated and flexion stretching exercises (knee-chest pulls, side bends, and pelvic rocks) are begun after the pain and inflammation have been substantially controlled.
6. Depending on the severity of the episode, crutches or a walker is strongly recommended as a transition to greater weightbearing after the obligate period of bed rest.
7. *Most common immobilizer:* A Velcro lumbosacral corset or sacroiliac belt is used for recurrent or chronic cases.

8. *Injection:* Local anesthesia can be used for differentiating sacroiliac symptoms from those that arise from the lower back and corticosteroid injection with triamcinolone acetonide 40 mg/mL (K40) for symptoms persisting beyond 6 weeks.
9. *Recovery exercises:* Flexion stretching exercises are combined with muscle toning exercises (modified sit-ups and weighted side bends) and general light aerobic exercise to complete the recovery.

SURGICAL PROCEDURE: None.

INJECTION: Local injection with anesthesia can be used to differentiate conditions affecting the sacroiliac joint from the local irritation and spasm of the paraspinal muscles (the origin of erector spinae), pain arising from the LS spine, or pain arising from the lower LS roots. Corticosteroid injection is used to treat the persistent inflammation of the sacroiliac joint that failed to respond to rest, physical therapy exercises, and bracing.

Positioning: The patient is placed in the prone position, perfectly flat.

Surface Anatomy and the Point of Entry: The PSIS is identified and marked. A line is drawn in the midline. The point of entry is 1 inch caudal to the PSIS and 1 inch lateral to the midline.

Angle of Entry and Depth: The angle of entry is 70 degrees with the needle directed outward. The depth of injection is $1\frac{1}{2}$ to $2\frac{1}{2}$ inches, depending on the weight of the patient.

Anesthesia: Ethyl chloride is sprayed on the skin. Ideally, 1 mL of local anesthesia is placed at the joint, i.e., the greatest possible depth. However, depending on the sensitivity of the patient, 0.5-mL-volume increments may need to be injected along the periosteum of the ileum or sacrum as the needle is advanced to the posterior aspect of the joint.

Technique: The successful injection of the sacroiliac joint requires a careful passage of the needle to the maximum depth allowable between the ileum and sacral bones (the sacrum and ileum form the sides of an inverted cone with the sacroiliac joint representing the apex). The needle is advanced down until the firm resistance of periosteum is encountered. If bone is encountered at

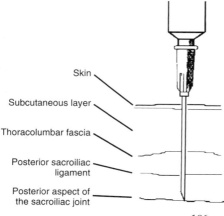

Skin
Subcutaneous layer
Thoracolumbar fascia
Posterior sacroiliac ligament
Posterior aspect of the sacroiliac joint

Figure 7-3B   Sacroiliac joint injection.

106

$1\frac{1}{2}$ inches, the needle is withdrawn 1 inch and redirected approximately 5 degrees and advanced until the maximum depth is achieved. If the injection is placed accurately, the local anesthetic effect should permit improved flexibility and decreased pain.

INJECTION AFTERCARE

1. The sacroiliac joint and the lower back must be *protected for the first 3 days* by avoiding direct pressure, bending, twisting, and all unnecessary walking and standing.
2. Three days of bed rest coupled with the use of crutches with touch-down weightbearing is strongly recommended for severe cases.
3. *Ice* (15 minutes every 4 to 6 hours), *acetaminophen* (1000 mg twice a day), or both, are used for postinjection soreness.
4. Movement of the back must be *limited* for 3 to 4 weeks by restricting prolonged standing, unnecessary walking, repetitive bending, lifting, and twisting.
5. A lumbosacral corset or sacral belt is prescribed for the first 2 to 3 weeks for recurrent or severe cases.
6. Passive *stretching exercises* of the back in flexion are begun when acute pain has begun to resolve (knee-chest pulls, pelvic rocks, and side bends).
7. The *injection* can be repeated at 6 weeks with corticosteroid if pain, inflammation, and secondary muscle spasm persist.
8. Active *toning exercises* of the abdominal and lower back muscle are begun only once flexibility has been restored.
9. *Plain film radiographs*, including oblique views, a standing anteroposterior pelvis for leg length discrepancy, a nuclear medicine bone scan, or *CT/MRI* is obtained to identify persistent sacroiliitis, short leg, sacral lesions, and so forth.

OUTCOME AND FURTHER WORK-UP: Isolated sacroiliac strain—unassociated with back or hip disease—has a favorable prognosis and responds well to local corticosteroid injection. Recurrent disease is either due to reinjury, associated conditions affecting the back and hip, or inflammatory sacroiliitis. Patients with multiple episodes of sacroiliac strain require a thorough examination of the lumbosacral spine and hip, plain films of the pelvis and lower back, and CT scanning or MRI of the lumbosacral spine. Patients with suspected sacroiliitis require blood work and a bone scan to determine the inflammatory activity.

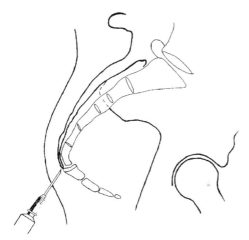

Enter 1 inch caudal to the sacrococcygeal junction in the midline; the needle is advanced at a 70-degree angle to the firm resistance of the posterior supporting ligaments or the hard resistance of bone
Needle: 1¹/₂-inch, 22-gauge
Depth: 1 to 1¹/₂ inches
Volume: 1 to 2 mL local anesthetic and 1 mL D80
NOTE: The injection should be placed flush against the supporting ligaments or the periosteum of the sacrum

Figure 7-4A   Injection of the sacrococcygeal junction for coccygodynia.

SUMMARY

Coccygodynia is an injury and subsequent inflammation of the articulation between the lowest sacral element and the coccyx. Patients complain of buttock pain aggravated by sitting or pain over the tailbone from any direct pressure. Examination demonstrates exquisite focal tenderness at the tail end of the spinal column in the midline. Most cases result either from blunt trauma (falls directly onto the edge of a stair, the edge of a chair, or an object on the ground) or as an aftermath of childbirth. The latter explains why nearly 90% are seen in young women. Patients more than 50 years of age who complain of pain in the buttock or tailbone area must undergo rectal and pelvic examinations to exclude anorectal or pelvic pathology.

TREATMENT OF CHOICE: Avoiding direct pressure is the single most important aspect of treatment.

SEQUENCE OF TREATMENTS
1. Ice may afford temporary relief but its application is impractical.
2. *Acute restrictions:* Avoiding direct pressure and the irritation of sitting, in particular, is the single most important restriction.
3. *Most common immobilizer:* A soft pillow, cushion, or hemorrhoidal pad is used to avoid direct pressure.
4. *Exercises of choice:* No specific exercises can reduce the pressure over the joint.
5. *Injection:* Local anesthetic can be used to confirm the diagnosis and corticosteroid injection with D80 used for symptoms persisting beyond 4 to 6 weeks.
6. *Recovery exercises:* Firming up the gluteus muscle with leg extension exercises may provide some protection against the direct pressure of sitting.

SURGICAL PROCEDURE: Coccygectomy is indicated when treatment fails, when symptoms persist, and especially if the sacrococcygeal junction has been fractured or otherwise altered from its normal round curvature.

INJECTION: Local injection with anesthetic can be used to differentiate conditions affecting the sacrococcygeal joint from the referred pain from the sacroiliac joint and from conditions affecting the rectum, lower colon, and pelvis. Corticosteroid injection is used to treat the persistent inflammation of the sacrococcygeal joint that fails to respond to rest, protection, and time.

Positioning: The patient is placed in the lateral decubitus position with the hips and knees flexed to 90 degrees, thus exposing the tail of the spine.

Surface Anatomy and the Point of Entry: The sacral prominence is identified and the gluteus crease is followed down to the inferior-most portion of the sacrum. Bimanual rectal examination can be used to define the exact location, the degree of sensitivity, and mobility of the sacrococcygeal joint. The point of entry is $\frac{1}{2}$ to 1 inch inferior to the joint in the midline.

Angle of Entry and Depth: The angle of entry is 70 degrees with the needle directed upward toward the sacrococcygeal joint. The depth of injection is $\frac{1}{2}$ to 1 inch, depending on the thickness of the subcutaneous layer.

Anesthesia: Ethyl chloride is sprayed on the skin; 0.5 mL of local anesthetic is placed just under the skin and another 0.5 to 1 mL is placed just adjacent to the joint.

Technique: The successful injection of the sacrococcygeal joint requires a careful passage of the needle to the firm resistance of the supporting ligaments or the hard resistance of the sacrum. An assistant is asked to place upward traction on the buttock to expose the gluteal crease. The examiner places one finger firmly against the lowest aspect of the sacrum. The point of entry is $\frac{1}{2}$ to 1 inch below the placement of the examiner's finger. After placing anesthesia in the subcutaneous tissue, the needle is advanced down to the supporting ligament or sacrum. Note that the joint is not actually entered. Another 0.5 mL of anesthetic is injected just outside this area. If the injection is placed accurately, the local anesthetic effect should reduce the pressure pain immediately; 1 mL of D80 is injected flush against the ligament or bone.

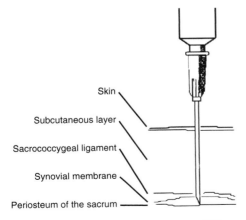

Skin

Subcutaneous layer

Sacrococcygeal ligament

Synovial membrane

Periosteum of the sacrum

Figure 7-4B   Coccygodynia injection.

INJECTION AFTERCARE

1. The sacrococcygeal joint must be ***protected for the first 3 days*** by avoiding direct pressure and all unnecessary sitting.
2. Three days of bed rest coupled with the use of crutches with touch-down weightbearing is strongly recommended for severe cases.
3. ***Acetaminophen*** (1000 mg twice a day) is used for postinjection soreness.
4. The joint must be ***protected*** for 3 to 4 weeks by limiting direct pressure and unnecessary sitting.
5. ***Most common immobilizer:*** A soft pillow, cushion, or hemorrhoidal pad is used to avoid direct pressure.
6. The ***injection*** can be repeated at 6 weeks with corticosteroid if pain and inflammation persist.
7. Active ***toning exercises*** of the gluteus muscles are begun only once pain and inflammation have significantly improved.
8. ***Plain film radiographs*** are obtained of the sacrum to evaluate angulation and irregularities of the joint and a ***consultation*** with an orthopedic surgeon can be considered for persistent pain and inflammation that fails to improve with two consecutive injections.

Chapter 8

HIP

THE DIFFERENTIAL DIAGNOSIS OF HIP PAIN

DIAGNOSES	CONFIRMATIONS
Hip bursa (most common)	
Trochanteric bursitis	Local anesthetic block
Gluteus medius bursitis	Local anesthetic block
Ischiogluteal bursitis	Local anesthetic block
Iliopectineal bursitis	Local anesthetic block
Snapping hip	Examination
Hip joint	
Osteoarthritis	Radiographs: standing anteroposterior pelvis
Inflammatory arthritis	Aspiration/synovial fluid analysis
Septic arthritis	Aspiration/synovial fluid analysis
Shallow acetabulum	Radiographs: standing
Subluxation/dislocation	anteroposterior pelvis
Hip prosthesis	
Loosening	Radiographs; bone scan
Prosthesis fracture	Radiographs: anteroposterior pelvis
Subluxation/dislocation	Radiographs: anteroposterior pelvis
Meralgia paresthetica	History; sensory examination
Bony pathology	
Avascular necrosis of the hip	Bone scan; magnetic resonance imaging (MRI)
Occult fracture of the hip	Bone scan; MRI
Malignancy	Bone scan; MRI
Referred pain	
Lumbosacral spine	Neurologic examination; computed tomography (CT) scanning
Sacroiliac joint	Radiographs; bone scanning
Vaso-occlusive disease	Examination; Doppler study
Inguinal hernia	Examination

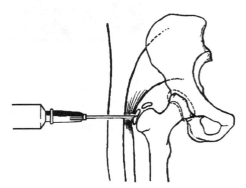

Enter over the midtrochanter in the lateral decubitus position; lightly advance the needle to the firm resistance of the gluteus medius tendon and then $\frac{1}{2}$ inch farther to the periosteum of the femur

Needle: $1\frac{1}{2}$-inch standard or $3\frac{1}{2}$-inch spinal needle, 22-gauge

Depth: $1\frac{1}{2}$ to 3 inches, down through the gluteus medius tendon to the periosteum

Volume: 1 to 2 mL local anesthetic and 1 mL K40

Figure 8-1A   Trochanteric bursa injection.

SUMMARY

Trochanteric bursitis is an inflammation of the lubricating sac located between the midportion of the trochanteric process of the femur and the gluteus medius tendon and the iliotibial tract. A disturbance in gait is implicated as the cause in 95% cases (arthritis, scoliosis, or disk disease in the lumbosacral spine, leg length discrepancy, sacroiliac strain, or the gait disturbance caused from a primary problem at the knee or ankle joint). Repetitive flexing at the hip and direct pressure aggravate this condition. Direct trauma to the outer thigh and osteoarthritis of the hip are relatively rare causes of this condition.

TREATMENT OF CHOICE: The cross-leg stretching exercise of the gluteus medius muscle combined with the specific treatment of the primary gait disturbance represents the initial treatment of choice.

SEQUENCE OF TREATMENTS

1. ***Exercise of choice:*** A properly performed cross-leg stretching exercise of the gluteus medius muscle lessens the pressure over the trochanteric bursa.
2. For the patient with severe pain or a severe disturbance of gait, touch-down weightbearing with crutches or a walker can be used for 5 to 7 days.
3. ***Acute restrictions:*** Direct pressure over the outer upper thigh and repetitive bending (stairs, bicycle, squatting, etc.) must be avoided by all patients.
4. Sitting and sleeping with the leg abducted to 45 degrees will reduce the pressure over the outer thigh.
5. A 3-week course of a nonsteroidal anti-inflammatory drug (NSAID) in full dose can be tried for mild to moderate cases.
6. ***Injection:*** Local corticosteroid injection with triamcinolone acetonide 40 mg/mL (K40) is indicated for severe symptoms lasting longer than 8 weeks (see details on page 113).
7. ***Recovery exercises:*** The flexion stretching exercises of the back (knee-chest pull, pelvic rocks, and side bends) combined with general aerobic conditioning complete the recovery.

SURGICAL PROCEDURE: Iliotibial tract release is performed for chronic bursitis that has failed to improve with exercise, with gait correction, and two or three injections performed over the course of the year. Bursectomy is rarely performed.

INJECTION: For an uncomplicated bursitis, local injection is the preferred anti-inflammatory treatment, especially if there is no obvious correctable underlying gait disturbance.

Positioning: The patient is placed in the lateral decubitus position with the affected side up and the knees flexed to 90 degrees (the trochanter is most prominent in this position).

Surface Anatomy and the Point of Entry: The superior, posterior, and anterior edges of the trochanteric process are palpated and marked. The point of entry is directly over the center point of the trochanter—$1\frac{1}{2}$ inches below the superior trochanter. Alternatively, the point of entry is at the crown of the trochanter, viewed tangentially in the anteroposterior (AP) and cephalad directions.

Angle of Entry and Depth: The needle is inserted perpendicularly to the skin. The depth is 1 to $2\frac{1}{2}$ inches to the gluteus medius and $1\frac{1}{2}$ to 3 inches to the femur (the gluteus medius tendon/iliotibial band is $\frac{3}{8}$ to $\frac{1}{2}$ inch thick).

Anesthesia: Ethyl chloride is sprayed on the skin. Local anesthetic is placed at the gluteus medius tissue plane (1 mL) and at the periosteum of the femur (0.5 mL).

Technique: The success of treatment depends on an accurate injection of the bursa at the level of the femur. The needle is held very lightly and advanced through the low resistance of the subcutaneous fat to the firm rubbery resistance of the gluteus medius tendon. Following anesthesia at this level, the needle is advanced (firm pressure) $\frac{1}{2}$ to $\frac{5}{8}$ inch farther to the periosteum of the femur. Caution: The patient will usually experience sharp pain as soon as the needle touches the periosteum! Injection at this deeper level requires firm pressure. If excessive pressure is encountered, the needle should be rotated 180 degrees or withdrawn ever so slightly. If the trochanter tenderness is significantly relieved, 1 mL of K40 is injected through the same needle.

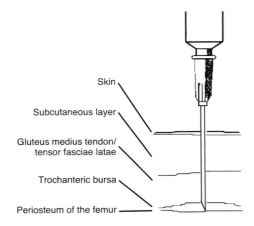

Skin

Subcutaneous layer

Gluteus medius tendon/
tensor fasciae latae

Trochanteric bursa

Periosteum of the femur

Figure 8-1B   Trochanteric bursa injection.

INJECTION AFTERCARE

1. The hip must be *protected for the first 3 days* by avoiding direct pressure and repetitive bending.
2. Three days of bed rest with the use of crutches with touch-down weightbearing is strongly recommended for severe cases.
3. *Ice* (15 minutes every 4 to 6 hours), *acetaminophen (Tylenol ES)* (1000 mg twice a day), or both, are used for postinjection soreness.
4. The hip must be *protected* for 3 to 4 weeks by limiting direct pressure and repetitive bending, prolonged standing, and unnecessary walking.
5. The cross-leg *stretching exercise* of the gluteus medius muscle is begun on day 4.
6. For those with accompanying structural back disease, passive *stretching exercises* of the lower back in flexion are begun after the acute pain has begun to resolve.
7. The *injection* can be repeated at 6 weeks with a corticosteroid if pain and inflammation persist.
8. *Plain film radiographs*, a standing AP pelvis for leg length discrepancy, a nuclear medicine bone scan, or *CT/MRI* is obtained to identify persistent, short leg, subtle disk, spondylolisthesis, and so forth.
9. Long-term restrictions of weightbearing and direct pressure are advised for the patient with chronic bursitis (5%).

OUTCOME AND FURTHER WORK-UP: Trochanteric bursitis responds dramatically to local corticosteroid injection. When combined with gluteus medius stretching and correction of the underlying gait disturbance, long-term benefits are expected. Patients with short-term benefits to treatment should be evaluated for chronic conditions affecting the lumbosacral spine, sacroiliac joint, leg length discrepancy, or functional or neurologic causes of high tension in the gluteus medius tendon (fibromyalgia, Parkinson's disease, residual tension from a previous stroke, etc.). Chronic bursitis develops in patients who have a refractory gait disturbance.

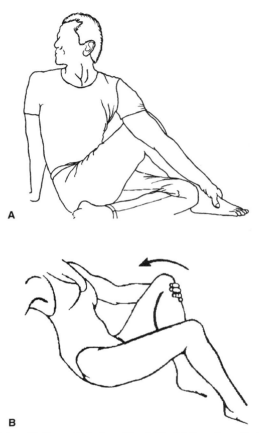

A

B

Figure 8-2 Gluteus Medius and Maximus Muscle Stretch Exercises—Stretching of the buttock tendons is used in the active treatment of trochanteric and gluteus medius bursitis and for the majority of conditions that affect the lower back (e.g., lumbosacral muscle strain, scoliosis, spondylolisthesis). These exercises are not only beneficial as a part of a comprehensive treatment plan but also can be prescribed for prevention of these same conditions. **A,** Cross-leg stretching exercise for gluteus medius. **B,** Knee-chest pull for gluteus maximus.

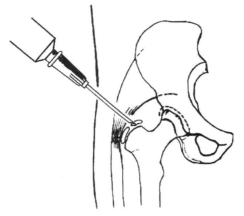

Enter 1 inch above the superior edge of the trochanteric process in the lateral decubitus position; advance the needle at a 45-degree angle down to the gluteus medius tendon and then to the periosteum of the femur

Needle: $1\frac{1}{2}$- to $3\frac{1}{2}$-inch spinal needle, 22-gauge

Depth: $1\frac{1}{2}$ to $3\frac{1}{2}$ inches (down to the periosteum)

Volume: 1 to 2 mL local anesthetic and 1 mL K40

Figure 8-3A   Injection of the gluteus medius bursa.

SUMMARY

Gluteus medius bursitis (also referred to as the "deep trochanteric bursa") is an inflammation of the bursal sac that is located between the superior portion of the trochanteric process and the gluteus medius tendon. It is identical to trochanteric bursitis in symptoms, presentation, underlying cause (primary gait disturbance), and treatment. It accompanies trochanteric bursitis in 30% of cases. The piriformis muscle attaches to the medial aspect of the superior trochanter (an abductor of the hip). Piriformis syndrome consists of pain about the hip, muscle spasm of the piriformis muscle, and a pain pattern that mimics sciatica (buttock pain that radiates down the leg caused by compression of the nerve as it courses thru the muscle).

TREATMENT OF CHOICE: Passive stretching exercises of the gluteus medius muscle and the iliotibial band (cross-leg stretching and lateral upper thigh stretching, respectively) are combined with the specific treatment of the primary gait disturbance.

SEQUENCE OF TREATMENTS

1. *Exercises of choice:* The cross-leg stretching exercise of the gluteus medius muscle and the upper thigh stretches of the iliotibial band combine to reduce the pressure over the outer hip.
2. Five to 7 days of touch-down weightbearing with crutches is recommended for patients with severe pain and a dramatic disturbance in gait,
3. *Acute restrictions:* Direct pressure over the outer hip, repetitive bending, prolonged standing, and unnecessary walking must be avoided.
4. Patients should be informed that sitting and sleeping with the leg abducted to 45 degrees will reduce the pressure over the outer hip.
5. A 3-week course of an NSAID is effective in mild to moderate cases.
6. *Injection:* Local corticosteroid injection with K40 is used in patients with symptoms lasting longer than 8 weeks (see details below).

116

7. **_Recovery exercises:_** Passive stretching exercises of the back in flexion (knee-chest pulls, pelvic rocks, and side bends) combined with general aerobic conditioning complete the treatment.

SURGICAL PROCEDURE: Iliotibial tract release is performed for chronic bursitis that has failed to improve with exercise, gait correction, and two or three injections performed over the course of the year. Bursectomy is rarely performed.

INJECTION: For an uncomplicated bursitis, that is, one not associated with a correctable underlying gait abnormality (mechanical low back stiffness, short leg, gait disturbance, etc.), local injection is the preferred treatment. Note: If both the gluteus and trochanteric bursa are involved, the trochanteric bursa should be treated first (the trochanteric bursa is the dominant bursa of the lateral hip).

Positioning: The patient is placed in the lateral decubitus position with the affected side up and the knees flexed to 90 degrees (the trochanter is most prominent in this position).

Surface Anatomy and the Point of Entry: The superior, posterior, and anterior edges of the trochanteric process are palpated and marked. The point of entry is $\frac{3}{4}$ to 1 inch above the midpoint of the superior-most portion of the trochanter. Alternatively, if the trochanteric process cannot be palpated directly, the superior point of entry can be identified by viewing the crown of the trochanter tangentially in the AP and cephalad directions.

Angle of Entry and Depth: The needle is inserted at a 45-degree angle in direct alignment with the femur. The depth is 1 to $2\frac{1}{2}$ inches to the gluteus medius tendon and $1\frac{1}{2}$ to 3 inches to the superior trochanter (the tendon is $\frac{1}{2}$ to $\frac{5}{8}$ inch thick).

Anesthesia: Ethyl chloride is sprayed on the skin. Local anesthetic is placed at the gluteus medius tendon (1 mL) and at the periosteum of the femur (0.5 mL).

Technique: The success of treatment depends on an accurate injection of the bursa at the level of the femur. The needle is held very lightly and advanced through the low resistance of the

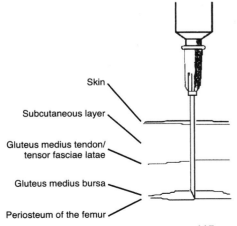

Skin

Subcutaneous layer

Gluteus medius tendon/
tensor fasciae latae

Gluteus medius bursa

Periosteum of the femur

Figure 8-3B Gluteus medius bursa injection.

subcutaneous fat to the firm rubbery resistance of the gluteus medius tissue plane. Following anesthesia at this level, the needle is advanced (firm pressure) $\frac{1}{2}$ to $\frac{5}{8}$ inch farther to the periosteum of the femur. Caution: The patient usually experiences sharp pain as soon as the needle touches the periosteum! Injection at this deeper level requires firm pressure. If excessive pressure is encountered, the needle should be rotated 180 degrees or withdrawn ever so slightly. If the local tenderness over the trochanter is significantly relieved, 1 mL of K40 is injected through the same needle.

INJECTION AFTERCARE
1. The hip must be *protected for the first 3 days* by avoiding direct pressure and repetitive bending.
2. Three days of bed rest with the use of crutches with touch-down weightbearing is strongly recommended for severe cases.
3. *Ice* (15 minutes every 4 to 6 hours), *acetaminophen* (1000 mg twice a day), or both, are used for postinjection soreness.
4. The hip must be *protected* for 3 to 4 weeks by limiting direct pressure and repetitive bending, prolonged standing, and unnecessary walking.
5. The cross-leg *stretching exercise* of the gluteus medius muscle is begun on day 4.
6. For those with accompanying structural back disease, passive *stretching exercises* of the lower back in flexion are begun after the acute pain has begun to resolve.
7. The *injection* can be repeated at 6 weeks with corticosteroid if pain and inflammation persist.
8. *Plain film radiographs*, a standing AP pelvis for leg length discrepancy, a nuclear medicine bone scan, or *CT/MRI* is obtained to identify persistent short leg, subtle disk, spondylolisthesis, and so forth.
9. Long term restrictions of weightbearing and direct pressure are advised for the patient with chronic bursitis (5%).

OUTCOME AND FURTHER WORK-UP: Trochanteric bursitis responds dramatically to local corticosteroid injection. When combined with gluteus medius stretching and correction of the underlying gait disturbance, long-term benefits are expected. Patients with short-term benefits from treatment should be evaluated for chronic conditions affecting the lumbosacral spine, sacroiliac joint, leg length discrepancy, or functional or neurologic causes of high tension in the gluteus medius tendon (fibromyalgia, Parkinson's disease, residual tension from a previous stroke, etc.). Chronic bursitis develops in patients who have a refractory gait disturbance.

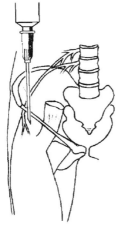

Enter 1 below and 1 inch medial to the anterior superior iliac spine (ASIS); advance the needle at a 90-degree angle down to the interface of the subcutaneous fat and the fascia of the quadriceps
Needle: $1\frac{1}{2}$-inch, 22-gauge
Depth: 1 to $1\frac{1}{2}$ inches (down to the fascia)
Volume: 1 to 2 mL local anesthetic and 1 mL K40

Figure 8-4A Injection of the lateral femoral cutaneous nerve.

SUMMARY

Meralgia paresthetica is a compression neuropathy of the lateral femoral cutaneous nerve as the nerve exits the pelvis, traverses the groin, and enters the thigh. The nerve penetrates the quadriceps fascia and enters the subcutaneous fat approximately 1 inch medial and 1 inch distal to the ASIS. This is the anatomic area where it is most vulnerable to the compressive forces of an overlying panniculus, tight garments worn around the waist, and scar tissue in and around the lateral aspect of the inguinal ligament. Changes on the neurologic examination are restricted to sensory abnormalities only (the nerve is a pure sensory nerve without a motor component). The degree of hypoesthesia (numbness and tingling) or hyperesthesia (burning quality pain) over the anterolateral aspect of the thigh varies according to the degree of nerve compression. In contrast with the spectrum of findings accompanying lumbar radiculopathy, the remainder of the neurologic examination (lower extremity reflexes, motor strength, muscle tone and bulk) and examination of the lower back is normal.

TREATMENT OF CHOICE: Any constriction around the waist must be avoided and the patient must be reassured that this isn't a pinched nerve from the back.

SEQUENCE OF TREATMENTS

1. The patient should be reassured that the condition is benign. (The nerve controlling the sensation of the thigh has been under pressure. As soon as the pressure is relieved, the feeling or irritative symptoms will gradually improve over several weeks.)
2. Tight garments around the waist must be avoided.
3. Ice is applied over the inguinal ligament and the ASIS to reduce irritation.
4. Weight loss must be emphasized in the obese patient.

5. ***Acute restrictions:*** Bending at the waist must be limited, especially if the patient has a large abdomen, and repetitive flexing of the hip should be avoided.
6. ***Exercises of choice:*** Abdominal toning exercises (half sit-ups, crunches, weighted side bends, etc.) cause a tightening of the inguinal area that in turn can reduce pressure over the nerve.
7. Severe cases with intractable dysesthetic pain can be treated with phenytoin (Dilantin) or carbamazepine (Tegretol).
8. ***Injection:*** Local anesthetic injection can be used to confirm the diagnosis and combined with corticosteroid to empirically treat the inflammation.
9. ***Consultation:*** Anesthesia consultation is recommended for possible nerve block.

SURGICAL PROCEDURE: Because most cases resolve with conservative treatment measures or time (91%), surgery is rarely necessary. For intractable dysesthetic pain, neurolysis of the constricting tissue, neurolysis and transposition of the nerve, or neurectomy can be performed.

INJECTION: Injection with anesthetic is used to confirm the diagnosis. Corticosteroid is used if symptoms persists for longer than 8 weeks despite restrictions and exercise.

Positioning: The patient is placed in the supine position with the legs keep straight.

Surface Anatomy and the Point of Entry: The ASIS is identified and marked. The inguinal ligament is identified as it courses to the lateral aspect of the pubic bone. The point of entry is $\frac{3}{4}$ to 1 inch medial to the ASIS and an equal distance below it midpoint of the superior-most portion of the trochanter.

Angle of Entry and Depth: The needle is inserted perpendicularly and advanced down to the firm tension of the fascia of the quadriceps femoris muscle. If an anesthetic block is not achieved at this point, the angle of entry is changed to a medially directed 45-degree angle. Similarly, if anesthetic block is not achieved at this point, the angle of entry is changed to a laterally directed 45-degree angle. In each case the depth of injection is just to the firm tension of the quadriceps femoris muscle

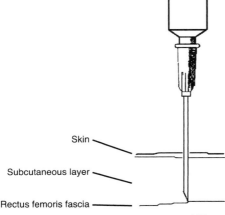

Skin

Subcutaneous layer

Rectus femoris fascia

Figure 8-4B   Meralgia paresthetica injection.

120

Anesthesia: Because of the variable entry point of the nerve into the anterior thigh—most enter medially to the ASIS and a minority enter either at the ASIS or just lateral to it—anesthetic is fanned out above the fascia to define its exact location. Precise corticosteroid injection requires an accurate localization of the lateral cutaneous femoral nerve. One to 2 mL is placed just above the fascia of quadriceps femoris muscle until anesthesia is achieved.

Technique: The success of treatment depends as much on the accurate localization of the lateral femoral cutaneous nerve by stepwise anesthetic block as on the placement of the corticosteroid just above the fascia and adjacent to the nerve. First, the level of the quadriceps muscle fascia is identified by gradually advancing the needle down until the firm resistance of the fascia is felt at the needle tip. If the fascia is not readily identified, applying skin traction in a back and forth manner will assist in defining the interface of the subcutaneous fat and the fascia. If the needle is above the fascia, the needle will move readily as traction is applied. If the needle has penetrated the fascia, the needle will not move in any direction when traction is applied. If the patient's symptoms are not reproduced by injecting above the fascia, the needle is withdrawn close to the surface of the skin and then reinserted at a 45-degree angle laterally or medially until an anesthetic block has been achieved. One or 2 mL of anesthetic is placed at each location and the patient is reexamined to evaluate its effectiveness. Once the location of the nerve has been identified, 1 mL of K40 is injected through the same needle.

INJECTION AFTERCARE

1. The anterior thigh must be ***protected for the first 3 days*** by avoiding direct pressure, repetitive bending, and repetitious flexing of the hip.
2. ***Ice*** (15 minutes every 4 to 6 hours), ***acetaminophen*** (1000 mg twice a day), or both, are used for postinjection soreness.
3. The anterior thigh must be ***protected*** for 3 to 4 weeks by limiting direct pressure and repetitive bending at the waist and repetitive flexing of the hip.
4. Attention to constricting garments at the waist and weight loss are continued.
5. The ***injection*** can be repeated at 6 weeks with corticosteroid if pain and inflammation persist.
6. ***CT/MRI*** is obtained if the patient's symptoms suggest a concomitant disk process in the upper lumbosacral spine area.
7. ***Consultation*** with a neurosurgeon can be considered for patients with intractable pain and those failing two injections over a period of several months.

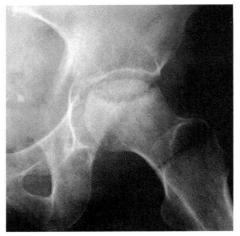

Ligamentum teres (blood supply to the
    proximal third of the head of the
    femur)
Femoral head
Developing fracture line
Femoral neck
Haversian canals in the femoral neck
    (blood supply to the distal two
    thirds of the head of the femur)

Figure 8-5   Avascular necrosis of the hip.

SUMMARY

Avascular necrosis of the hip results from an interruption of the normal blood supply to the proximal portion of the femoral head. Common causes include trauma, diabetes, alcoholism, high viscosity hematologic states, and oral corticosteroids (especially in young asthmatic, rheumatoid arthritic, or lupus patients). Early diagnosis is elusive because of the nonspecific presenting complaints and physical signs. The diagnosis should be suspected if (1) the patient is at risk, (2) anterior groin pain is acute and dramatic, (3) weightbearing causes severe pain, and (4) rotation of the hip causes severe pain. Note that radiographs of the hip obtained in the first week or two are usually normal.

TREATMENT OF CHOICE: Non-weightbearing with crutches or a walker is mandatory until the diagnosis is either made or excluded by special testing.

SEQUENCE OF TREATMENTS

1. *Acute restriction:* Non-weightbearing with crutches is preferred in hope of preventing collapse of the avascular segment.
2. MRI is the test of choice to evaluate for a fracture line at the proximal third of the femoral head.
3. Laboratory testing should evaluate the general health of the patient and look for underlying risk factors. These should include the following: complete blood count (CBC), erythrocyte sedimentation rate (ESR), glucose, liver function test (LFT), serum protein electrophoresis (SPEP), calcium, and alkaline phosphatase.
4. *Consultation:* Orthopedic referral to assist in the management is advised.
5. If special studies are not available, ***plain film radiographs*** can be repeated in 2 to 3 weeks.

6. *Recovery exercises:* Range of motion exercises are combined with progressive ambulation. Weightbearing is permitted when rotation of the hip is no longer painful and healing has been clearly demonstrated on plain film radiographs.

SURGICAL PROCEDURE: Core decompression is performed before the collapse of the fracture segment. Total hip replacement is the procedure of choice when femoral head collapse (coxa plana) has occurred.

OUTCOME AND FURTHER WORK-UP: The outcome of avascular necrosis depends on making the diagnosis in a timely fashion, protecting the fracture segment from collapse by avoiding weightbearing, and to a certain extent, luck. MRI is always indicated as is a full laboratory work-up. The primary care provider should work together with the orthopedic surgeon in evaluating the patient.

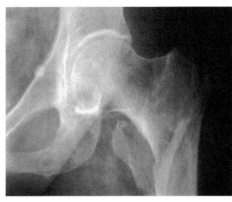

Occult fracture of the hip must be
suspected if:
1. A fall has occurred in an elderly
   patient with known osteoporotic
   bones
2. Weightbearing is impossible
   because of moderate to severe hip
   pain
3. Internal and external rotation of the
   hip causes moderate to severe hip
   pain on examination
NOTE: Plain film radiographs of the
   hip do not demonstrate a true
   fracture

Figure 8-6 Proper management of occult fracture of the hip should prevent progression to complete fracture.

SUMMARY

The diagnosis of hip fracture is usually obvious based on a history of injury, the foreshortened and externally rotated leg, and the typical changes on plain film radiographs. However, an incomplete or greenstick fracture of the femur may elude early detection because of the history of a trivial fall, the lack of typical changes on examination, the difficulties in interpreting plain films with advanced osteoporosis, and the nondisplaced nature of the fracture. The diagnosis should be suspected when weightbearing is associated with apprehension or dramatic pain and the examination of the hip discloses severe pain and extreme guarding with rotation of the hip. Plain film radiographs are not reliable in the presence of dramatic degrees of osteopenia. Medicolegally, this condition must be treated with non-weightbearing in order to avoid the risk of litigation if the unprotected hip progresses to complete fracture!

TREATMENT OF CHOICE: Non-weightbearing with crutches or a walker is mandatory until the diagnosis is either confirmed or excluded by special testing.

SEQUENCE OF TREATMENTS
1. *Acute restriction:* Non-weightbearing with crutches or bed rest is absolutely necessary.
2. MRI is used to evaluate for occult fracture.
3. *Consultation:* Referral to an orthopedic surgery is strongly advised.
4. If special studies are not available, *plain film radiographs* can be repeated in 2 to 3 weeks to look for signs of healing (however, the patient must be kept non-weightbearing through this interval).
5. *Recovery exercises:* Range of motion exercises are combined with progressive ambulation. Weightbearing is allowed when rotation of the hip is free from pain and significant healing has been demonstrated on plain film radiographs.

SURGICAL PROCEDURE: The choice between hip pinning or total hip replacement depends on the type and severity of the fracture, the general health and condition of the patient, and the patient's age.

Chapter 9

KNEE

THE DIFFERENTIAL DIAGNOSIS OF KNEE PAIN

DIAGNOSES	CONFIRMATIONS
Patella (most common)	
Subluxation/dislocation	Examination; radiographs: sunrise views
Patellofemoral syndrome	Examination; radiographs: sunrise views
Dashboard knee (chondral fracture)	Arthroscopy (optional)
Patellofemoral osteoarthritis	Radiographs: sunrise views
Patella alta	Radiographs: lateral view of the knee
Main joint	
Osteoarthritis: medial compartment, lateral compartment, or both	Radiographs: bilateral standing, anteroposterior (AP) knees
Inflammatory arthritis	Aspiration/synovial fluid analysis
Septic arthritis	Aspiration/synovial fluid analysis
Hemarthrosis	Aspiration/synovial fluid analysis
Bursa	
Prepatellar bursitis ("housemaid's knee")	Aspiration/bursal fluid analysis
Anserine bursitis	Local anesthetic block
Baker's cyst	Aspiration or ultrasound
Infrapatellar (superficial or deep)	Local anesthetic block
Ligaments	
Medial collateral injury: first, second, third	Examination; anesthetic block
Lateral collateral injury: first, second, third	Examination; local anesthetic block
Anterior cruciate injury	Examination; magnetic resonance imaging (MRI)
Posterior cruciate injury	Examination; MRI
Meniscal tear	
Traumatic or degenerative	MRI; arthroscopy
Iliotibial band syndrome	
Snapping knee	Examination; local anesthetic block
	Examination
Referred pain	
Trochanteric bursitis	Examination; local anesthetic block
Hip joint	Radiographs: standing AP pelvis
Femur	Bone scan
Lumbosacral spine radiculopathy	Computed tomography scan; MRI; electromyogram

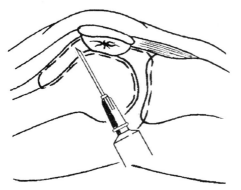

The patellofemoral family of
conditions include patellofemoral
syndrome, patellofemoral
subluxation, patellofemoral arthritis,
patellar dislocation, and patella alta
All of these are characterized by
abnormal tracking of the patella in
the femoral groove
Intra-articular corticosteroid injection
is indicated in patients with
refractory symptoms and the rare
patient with joint effusion

Figure 9-1   Injection of the knee for patellofemoral syndrome.

SUMMARY

The patellofemoral conditions consist of a group of similar conditions that cause symptoms at the patellofemoral joint, including patellofemoral syndrome (formally chondromalacia patella, the term describing the pathology), patellar subluxation (the mechanical term describing the abnormal tracking), patella alta (abnormal length of the patellar tendon), and patellofemoral arthritis (the end result of years of abnormal tracking). Although some cases are caused by direct trauma (dashboard knee), most of the patellofemoral conditions are a result of abnormal tracking of the patella in the femoral groove—patellar subluxation. An overdeveloped vastus lateralis muscle (a lack of balance with the weaker vastus medialis) and the Q angle formed by the tibial tubercle, the center of the patella, and the center of the quadriceps muscle create the forces that cause lateral patellar subluxation. Clinical findings include anteromedial pain caused by medial retinacular traction, retropatellar crepitation, anterior patellar clicking, and subluxation on the sunrise view of the knee.

TREATMENT OF CHOICE: The isometrically performed straight-leg-raise exercise with the leg externally rotated and in full extension enhances the tone of the vastus medialis and serves to counteract the lateral forces applied to the patella.

SEQUENCE OF TREATMENTS

1. Ice placed over the anterior knee is an effective analgesic.
2. *Acute restrictions:* Squatting or kneeling must be avoided. Repetitive flexion must be restricted according to the severity of the condition (to 30 degrees for severe disease or to 60 degrees for moderate disease).
3. *Exercises of choice:* The straight-leg-raise exercise with the lower leg externally rotated and in full extension is used to enhance the tone of the vastus medialis.
4. A 3-week course of a nonsteroidal anti-inflammatory drug (NSAID) can be tried, noting that this condition is more mechanical than inflammatory.
5. *Most common immobilizer:* A Velcro patellar restraining brace or patellar strap holds the patella in the femoral groove, thereby improving patellofemoral tracking.

6. ***Injection:*** Either hyaluronic acid injection or corticosteroid injection with triamcinolone acetonide 40 mg/mL (K40) is used for symptoms lasting longer than 8 weeks or for those patients who exhibit an associated joint effusion (see details on pages 129-130).
7. ***Recovery exercises:*** The straight-leg-raise exercise combined with hamstring leg extensions is used to complete the recovery.
8. ***Consultation:*** Patients with persistent symptoms, patellofemoral disease with Q angles more than 20 degrees, or recurrent patellar dislocation can be considered for orthopedic consultation.

SURGICAL PROCEDURE: Lateral retinacular release, tibial tubercle transposition, or arthroscopic débridement are the most common procedures performed.

INJECTION: Hyaluronic acid injection should be used for patients exhibiting chronic mechanical symptoms of pain, crepitation, and clicking, which respond more predictably to the injection. Patients with more inflammatory symptoms—intractable pain, persistent effusion, and poor responses to exercise and the NSAIDs—should be treated with corticosteroid injection. For the technique of intra-articular injection, see pages 129-130.

OUTCOME AND FURTHER WORK-UP: The prognosis of patellofemoral syndrome—the most common diagnosis in young and middle-aged adults—is uniformly good. The condition is rarely disabling and rarely remains symptomatic beyond age 50. Symptoms can wax and wane over many years, but the natural history of the condition for most is to gradually fade in the fifth decade. Patients with frequently recurring or severe symptoms should have repeat bilateral sunrise radiographs, synovial fluid analysis, or arthroscopy to evaluate for osteochondritis dissecans, inflammatory effusion, focal chondromalacia, and so forth.

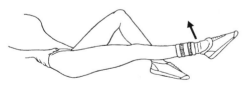

Figure 9-2   The Straight-Leg-Raise Exercise for Isometric Toning of the Quadriceps—This is the universal knee exercise used in the rehabilitation of the knee. It can be considered the treatment of choice in nearly all the conditions that affect the knee with the exception of the acute unstable bony fracture and the severe grade 3 ligament tears. Loss of quadriceps and hamstring muscle tone compromises the stability of the joint (the patient often complains of "giving out," a sense of looseness, and weak legs). Restoration or enhancement of the anterior and posterior thigh muscles tightens the joint, likely assists in the reabsorption of excess joint fluid, and reduces the chance of further injury to the articular cartilage and supporting structures. This exercise should be performed once or twice a day.

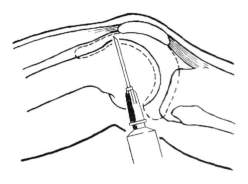

Enter laterally between the lines
formed by the underside of the
patella and the middle of the
iliotibial track; gently advance the
needle to the mild resistance of the
lateral retinaculum, angling just
above the superior pole of the
patella
Needle: $1\frac{1}{2}$- to $3\frac{1}{2}$-inch spinal needle,
22- to 18-gauge
Depth: $\frac{1}{2}$ to 3 inches
Volume: 1 to 2 mL anesthetic and
1 mL K40
NOTE: The synovial cavity is $\frac{1}{2}$ to $\frac{5}{8}$
inch beyond the lateral retinaculum;
aspirate with mild pressure as the
needle is advanced to this depth

Figure 9-3A   Intra-articular injection of knee by the lateral approach entering the suprapatellar pouch.

SUMMARY

A knee effusion is an abnormal accumulation of synovial fluid. It is classified as hemorrhagic, noninflammatory, inflammatory, or septic, depending on the cellular content (see synovial fluid table, page 210 in the appendix). Osteoarthritis, inflammatory arthritis, hemarthrosis due to trauma, and infection (gonococcus, *Staphylococcus*, and so forth) are the most common causes. Increasing amounts of fluid interfere with the normal movement of the knee, initially restricting flexion but eventually interfering with full extension. In addition, the hydraulic pressure of repetitive bending forces the synovial fluid into the popliteal space, causing the symptom of posterior tightness, impairment of flexion, and the formation of a Baker's cyst (approximately 10% to 15% of cases). Large effusions stretch the supporting structures surrounding the knee, contributing to ligament instability.

TREATMENT OF CHOICE: Aspiration and drainage of the synovial fluid is the treatment of choice for knee effusions associated with the persistent pain, loss of full flexion, repeated episodes of giving out, and instability (traumatic hemarthrosis and the large, tense effusions of acute arthritis). Aspiration, synovial fluid analysis, and corticosteroid injection are the treatments of choice for the nonseptic effusion.

SEQUENCE OF TREATMENTS

1. Immediate aspiration of fluid using an 18- to 20-gauge needle on a 20-mL syringe is used for hemarthrosis, tense effusions, and undiagnosed effusions. Synovial fluid is analyzed for cell count, crystals, differential, Gram stain and culture and sensitivity (C/S), and hematocrit (Hct) (see synovial fluid table, page 210 in the appendix).
2. Ice placed over the anterior knee is an effective analgesic and helps to reduce swelling.
3. *Acute restrictions:* Squatting and kneeling must be avoided. Flexion of the knee must be restricted according to the degree of the problem (to 30 degrees for severe disease or 60 degrees for moderate disease).

128

4. ***Exercises of choice:*** The straight-leg-raise exercise is used to restore muscle support, enhance stability, and reduce recurrent effusion.
5. A 3-week course of an NSAID in full dosage is an effective treatment.
6. ***Most common immobilizers:*** A neoprene pull-on brace or Velcro patellar restraining brace can be used for 2 to 3 weeks, but only until the quadriceps muscle tone is restored.
7. ***Injection:*** Corticosteroid injection with K40 is indicated when symptoms persist beyond 8 weeks.
8. ***MRI*** is indicated to further evaluate patients with persistent effusions, especially those patients presenting with mechanical symptoms, hemarthrosis, and with a poor response to injection.
9. ***Consultation:*** Orthopedic consultation is recommended for persistent symptoms related to advanced osteoarthritis, meniscal tear, loose body, and so forth.
10. ***Recovery exercises:*** The straight-leg-raise exercise combined with hamstring leg extensions will complete the recovery.

SURGICAL PROCEDURE: The choice of the surgical procedure depends on the diagnosis, length of symptoms, poor response to medical treatment, and so forth. Arthroscopic débridement, meniscectomy, and synovectomy are the most common procedures.

INJECTION: Aspiration of synovial fluid is performed to relieve the pressure of tense effusions and obtain fluid for analysis. The injection of local anesthetic can be used to differentiate the involvement of the joint from involvement of the soft tissues (bursa, tendon, etc.). Corticosteroid injection is used to treat the nonseptic effusion (osteoarthritis, rheumatoid arthritis, pseudogout, etc.).

Positioning: The patient is placed in the supine position with the leg fully extended. A rolled-up towel is placed under the knee if full extension is uncomfortable. The patient must be able to relax the quadriceps muscle.

Surface Anatomy and the Point of Entry: The midline of the iliotibial band, the lateral edge of the patella, and the superior pole of the patella are palpated and marked. The patella is gently pushed laterally to palpate its edge. The point of entry is along a line drawn halfway between the

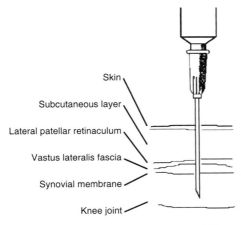

Skin

Subcutaneous layer

Lateral patellar retinaculum

Vastus lateralis fascia

Synovial membrane

Knee joint

Figure 9-3B   Intra-articular injection of knee.

129

iliotibial band (the center of the femur) and the lateral edge of the patella and $\frac{1}{2}$ inch below the superior pole of the patella (see Fig. 9-3A).

Angle of Entry and Depth: The needle is angled up toward the superior pole of the patella. The lateral retinaculum (first tissue plane) is between $\frac{1}{2}$ and $2\frac{1}{2}$ inches deep, depending on the thickness of the dermis. The superior pouch of the synovial cavity is always $\frac{1}{2}$ to $\frac{5}{8}$ inch beyond the lateral retinaculum.

Anesthesia: Ethyl chloride is sprayed on the skin. Local anesthetic is placed at the retinaculum (1 mL) and intra-articularly.

Technique: A **lateral approach** to the suprapatellar pouch is most accessible, closer to the skin, and less likely to cause painful irritation. The needle is advanced at a 70-degree angle toward the superior pole of the patella until the rubbery tissue resistance of the lateral retinaculum is felt; 1 mL of anesthetic is placed just outside this first tissue plane. The needle is withdrawn. Next, an 18-gauge $1\frac{1}{2}$-inch needle attached to a 20-mL syringe is advanced down to the retinaculum and then into the joint (a "giving way" sensation or pop is often felt and the patient may feel discomfort). To assist in aspirating fluid, gentle pressure against the medial retinaculum and joint line may shift the synovial fluid laterally. If the fluid is relatively clear (the examiner should be able to read newsprint through a low cell count fluid), 1 mL of K40 is injected through the same needle. If the first pass into the joint does not yield synovial fluid, the needle is slowly withdrawn with constant low suction. If fluid is not obtained with the slow withdrawal of the needle, the needle is redirected to the level of the superior pole of the patella. Aspiration is attempted at this site. If the second attempt is unsuccessful, a dry tap knee injection is recommended (see page 132).

INJECTION AFTERCARE

1. The knee must be **protected for the first 3 days** by avoiding direct pressure, squatting, kneeling, and bending beyond 90 degrees.
2. Crutches with touch-down weightbearing for 3 to 7 days are strongly advised for severe cases.
3. **Ice** (15 minutes every 4 to 6 hours), **acetaminophen (Tylenol ES)** (1000 mg twice a day), or both, are used for postinjection soreness.
4. The knee must be **protected** for 3 to 4 weeks by limiting direct pressure and repetitive bending, prolonged standing, and unnecessary walking; continue to restrict squatting and kneeling.
5. **Straight-leg-raise exercises** of the quadriceps muscle are begun on day 4 to enhance the support of the knee.
6. For those patients with poor quadriceps muscle tone or those patients with frequent giving out of the knee, temporary bracing (3 to 4 weeks) with a patellar restraining brace or even a Velcro straight leg brace is recommended.
7. The **injection** can be repeated at 6 weeks with corticosteroid if pain and swelling persist.
8. **Plain film radiographs** (standing posterolateral knees, bilateral sunrise views) or **MRI** is obtained in the chronic case to identify advanced degenerative arthritis, high degree subluxation of the patellofemoral joint, degenerative or traumatic meniscal tear, and so forth.
9. Long-term restrictions of bending (30 to 45 degrees) and the impact of weightbearing are advised for the patient with chronic symptoms.
10. Request a **consultation** for a second opinion with a surgical orthopedist if two consecutive injections fail to provide 4 to 6 months of improved function and decreased swelling.

OUTCOME AND FURTHER WORK-UP: The need for further work-up is determined by the response to corticosteroid injection. Further testing is usually unnecessary in patients with pseudogout, gout, and acute rheumatoid arthritis that respond dramatically. Patients with osteoarthritis often have associated anserine bursitis, medial collateral ligament (MCL) strain, or degenerative meniscal tears. And although they respond to injection, these associated conditions require follow-up, reevaluation, and treatment. However, patients who experience only a short-term (days) response require a thorough work-up. The failure to resolve the acute pain and swelling suggests the primary diagnosis affecting the knee is more of a mechanical rather than an inflammatory-based process. Further work-up should include repeat bilateral weightbearing radiographs, MRI, bone scan, or arthroscopy to evaluate for meniscal tear, anterior cruciate ligament (ACL) insufficiency, loose body, or failed or extremely injured articular cartilage. Obviously a successful outcome is rewarding. However, a limited response to injection is just as important because it identifies patients needing further testing!

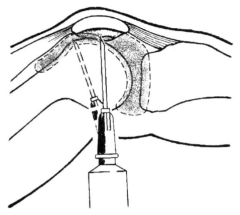

The same point of entry for aspiration of a knee effusion (page 128) is used for this injection; direct the needle toward the under surface of the patella

Needle: $1\frac{1}{2}$- to $3\frac{1}{2}$-inch spinal needle, 18- to 22-gauge

Depth: $\frac{1}{2}$ to 3 inches until the soft resistance of the patellar cartilage is felt

Volume: 1 to 2 mL anesthetic and 1 mL K40

Figure 9-4A   Dry tap intra-articular injection of knee by the lateral approach to the patella.

SUMMARY

Because the first attempt to obtain synovial fluid from a lateral approach to the suprapatellar pouch was unsuccessful, an alternative method is necessary to guarantee an intra-articular placement of medication; hence, the dry tap injection against the underside of the patella. If the tip of the needle is resting next to articular cartilage, an intra-articular injection is guaranteed.

Positioning: The patient is placed in the supine position with the leg fully extended.

Surface Anatomy and the Point of Entry: The midline of the iliotibial band, the lateral edge of the patella, and the superior pole of the patellar are palpated and marked. The patella should be gently moved laterally to palpate its lateral edge. The point of entry in the horizontal plane is halfway between the iliotibial band and the lateral edge of the patella and $\frac{1}{2}$ inch caudal to the superior pole of the patella in the craniocaudal axis.

Angle of Entry and Depth: The needle is angled up toward the under surface of the patella. The lateral retinaculum (first tissue plane) ranges from $\frac{1}{2}$ to $2\frac{1}{2}$ inches deep. The articular cartilage of the patella is $\frac{1}{2}$ to $\frac{3}{4}$ inch beyond the firm tissue resistance of the retinaculum.

Anesthesia: Ethyl chloride is sprayed on the skin. Local anesthetic is placed at the retinaculum (1 mL) and intra-articularly.

Technique: A **lateral approach** is easiest and safest. The same point of entry used for the lateral approach to the suprapatellar pouch (see page 129) is used to perform the dry tap injection. The needle is directed and advanced to the under surface of the patella. Mild subluxation of the patella will facilitate this injection. Firm pressure is necessary to pop into the joint. The bevel of the needle should be turned up so that the angle of the patella matches the bevel (this is less likely to damage the articular cartilage!). Then the needle is advanced cautiously to the under surface of the patella. The proper depth of injection is assessed by gently rocking the patella back and forth. Pressure applied along the medial edge of the patella should be felt at the tip of the needle. Be

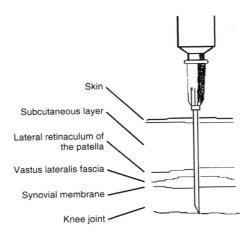

Skin

Subcutaneous layer

Lateral retinaculum of
the patella

Vastus lateralis fascia

Synovial membrane

Knee joint

Figure 9-4B   Dry tap injection of the knee.

extremely careful to avoid moving the tip of the needle back and forth when making contact with the cartilage of the patella. At this exact point, 1 to 2 mL of anesthetic can be injected (diagnostic local anesthetic block for an intra-articular process) along with either 2 mL of hyaluronic acid or 1 mL of K40.

INJECTION AFTERCARE
1. The knee must be *protected for the first 3 days* by avoiding direct pressure, all squatting, kneeling, and bending beyond 90 degrees.
2. Crutches with touch-down weightbearing for 3 to 7 days are strongly advised for severe cases.
3. *Ice* (15 minutes every 4 to 6 hours), *acetaminophen* (1000 mg twice a day), or both, are used for postinjection soreness.
4. The knee must be *protected* for 3 to 4 weeks by limiting direct pressure and repetitive bending, prolonged standing, and unnecessary walking; continue to restrict squatting and kneeling.
5. *Straight-leg-raise exercises* of the quadriceps muscle are begun on day 4 to enhance support of the knee.
6. For those patients with poor quadriceps muscle tone or with frequent giving out of the knee, temporary bracing (3 to 4 weeks) with a patellar restraining brace or even a Velcro straight leg brace is recommended.
7. The *injection* can be repeated at 6 weeks with corticosteroid if pain and swelling persist.
8. *Plain film radiographs* (standing PA knees, bilateral sunrise views) or *MRI* is obtained in the chronic case to identify advanced degenerative arthritis, high degree subluxation of the patellofemoral joint, degenerative or traumatic meniscal tear, and so forth.
9. Long-term restrictions of bending (30 to 45 degrees) and the impact of weightbearing are advised for the patient with chronic symptoms.
10. Request a *consultation* for a second opinion with a surgical orthopedist if two consecutive injections fail to provide 4 to 6 months of improved function and decreased swelling.

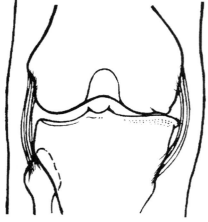

Medial joint narrowing (normally 6 to 8 mm)
Bone spur, squared off tibial plateau
Tibial plateau sclerosis
Angulation of the tibia and femur (normally 8 to 10 degrees of valgus)

Figure 9-5   Wear-and-tear arthritis of the knee.

SUMMARY

Osteoarthritis of the knee is a wear-and-tear mildly inflammatory arthritis that affects the three compartments of the joint—medial, lateral, and patellofemoral. A family history, obesity, genu valgum and genu varum, previous meniscectomy, and previous fractures of the distal femur and proximal tibia predispose to this condition. Pathologically, there is asymmetric wear of the articular cartilage, bony osteophyte formation, sclerosis of the subchondral bone, and subchondral cyst formation. Radiographically, a standing radiograph of the knee demonstrates a narrowing of the articular cartilage between the tibia and the femur. Involvement of the medial compartment predominates given the center of gravity is medially to the knee. Isolated involvement of the lateral compartment suggests previous injury either to the meniscal cartilage or the supporting ligaments

TREATMENT OF CHOICE: The straight-leg-raise exercise performed isometrically is the treatment of choice along with restrictions of use.

SEQUENCE OF TREATMENTS

1. Ice over the anterior knee is an effective analgesic and aids in reducing swelling.
2. *Acute restrictions:* Squatting and kneeling must be avoided and repetitive bending is restricted according to the severity of the condition (to 30 degrees for severe disease or to 60 degrees for moderate disease).
3. *Exercise of choice:* Isometric straight-leg-raise exercises are performed daily to restore or enhance the tone of the quadriceps muscle.
4. A 3-week course of an NSAID in full dose is effective in mild to moderate cases.
5. *Most common immobilizer:* A temporary (3 to 4 weeks) Velcro patellar restraining brace or Velcro straight leg brace is used until quadriceps tone is restored.

6. ***Injection:*** Local injection of corticosteroid with K40 or hyaluronic acid is indicated for arthritic flares lasting longer than 8 weeks and for persistent joint effusion (see details pages 129-130).
7. ***Consultation:*** Orthopedic consultation can be considered for patients that fail to experience at least 6 months of relief with either injections with corticosteroid and hyaluronic acid, for persistent loss of ambulatory function, or for patients that have signs and symptoms of a degenerative meniscal tear.
8. ***Recovery exercises:*** Straight-leg-raise exercises are combined with hamstring leg extensions to complete the recovery.

SURGICAL PROCEDURE: Surgery is indicated for advanced disease. Arthroscopic débridement is indicated for degenerative meniscal tears and loose bodies. High tibial osteotomy is the procedure of choice for patients younger than age 62 to correct the loss of normal 8- to 9-degree valgus angle and to shift the patient's weightbearing over to the preserved articular cartilage of the lateral compartment. Total knee replacement (TKR) is typically reserved for patients older than the age of 62 with bone-on-bone advanced disease.

INJECTION: Local corticosteroid or hyaluronic acid injection can provide dramatic short-term relief and is indicated when (1) NSAIDs are contraindicated, (2) NSAIDs are poorly tolerated, (3) inflammation and effusion fail to improve, (4) palliation is necessary for a patient who has advanced disease and cannot undergo surgery, or (5) the patient prefers it (see pages 129-130). Note that a lateral approach for aspiration and injection may not be suitable for all patients, especially those with severe hypertrophic patellofemoral disease. In these cases, a medial approach can be performed that is analogous to the lateral approach. The point of entry is halfway between the medial edge of the patella and the midplane of the leg (the center point of the femur).

OUTCOME AND FURTHER WORK-UP: Osteoarthritis can be complicated by effusion, anserine bursitis, MCL strain, or degenerative meniscal tears. Patients with osteoarthritis and an associated effusion respond predictably to injection. Patients with partial responses to injection often have an associated bursitis, ligament injury, or meniscal tear. These patients require follow-up examination, reevaluation of the original signs, and appropriate treatment. However, patients who experience a short-term (days) response require further testing with repeat bilateral, weightbearing radiographs, MRI, bone scan, or arthroscopy to evaluate for meniscal tear, ACL insufficiency, loose body, or failed or extremely injured articular cartilage.

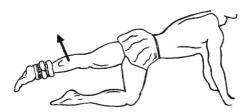

Figure 9-6   Leg Extensions for Isometric Toning of the Hamstring Muscles—This exercise is intended to balance the strength of the quadriceps muscle. A set of 20 repetitions, each held 5 seconds, is performed daily. Initially these are performed with just the weight of the leg; 5- to 10-pound weights are added as the strength and endurance of the muscles improves. This exercise should be performed lying prone if the patient experiences pain with direct pressure over the patella.

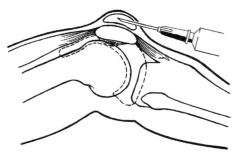

The bursa is entered at the base, parallel the patella; the needle is passed into the center of the sac; alternatively, the needle can be advanced to the lower third of the periosteum of the patella for injection of the small or chronically thickened bursa

Needle: $1\frac{1}{2}$-inch, 18- to 22-gauge

Depth: $\frac{1}{4}$ to $\frac{3}{8}$ inch

Volume: 1 to 2 mL anesthetic and 1 mL K40

NOTE: Placement of the needle on the periosteum guarantees an intrabursal injection

Figure 9-7A   Aspiration and injection of the prepatellar bursa.

SUMMARY

Prepatellar bursitis is an inflammation of the bursal sac located between the patella and the overlying skin. Most cases result from direct trauma as in a fall onto the knee or from the direct pressure and friction of repetitive kneeling (90% housemaid's knee). It is one of two bursae in the body that can become infected (5% due to staphylococci) or inflamed by urate crystals (5% due to acute gout). Normally the bursa is a paper-thin, fluid-filled potential space. With chronic irritation and inflammation, the bursal walls dilate, thicken, and eventually undergo fibrosis, the pathologic condition of chronic bursitis.

TREATMENT OF CHOICE: In order to define the exact cause of the bursal swelling, aspiration and laboratory testing of the fluid are necessary. Complete drainage of the distended bursa facilitates resolution and reduces the chance of recurrent and chronic bursitis.

SEQUENCE OF TREATMENTS

1. *Injection:* Aspiration, drainage, and fluid analysis are strongly recommended (see details on page 137).
2. *Most common immobilizer:* A compression dressing is applied immediately after the procedure and left in place for 36 to 48 hours, followed by a neoprene pull-on brace.
3. Ice over the anterior knee is an effective analgesic and helps to reduce swelling.
4. *Restrictions:* Direct pressure (kneeling or squatting) must be absolutely avoided and bending must be limited to 90 degrees.
5. Antibiotics are begun immediately if infection is documented on Gram stain or is suspected clinically; intravenous antibiotics are necessary if cellulitis accompanies septic bursitis.
6. If uric acid or calcium hydroxyapatite crystals are demonstrated, a 10-day course of an NSAID in full dose is prescribed.
7. *Exercise of choice:* Isometric straight-leg-raise exercises are performed if decreased activity has reduced quadriceps muscle tone.
8. *Aspiration* can be repeated at 4 to 6 weeks and combined with an *injection* of K40 if fluid reaccumulates at this early interval.
9. Repeat the aspiration and local corticosteroid injection for a second recurrence.

10. ***Recovery exercises:*** Straight-leg-raise exercises are combined with hamstring leg extensions for general conditioning of the knee.
11. ***Consultation:*** Surgical consultation is recommended for symptoms that fail to be controlled by two consecutive injections.
12. Patients whose occupations require constant kneeling or squatting must be advised of the possibility of recurrence and strongly encouraged to wear a protective kneepad.

SURGICAL PROCEDURE: Bursectomy is infrequently performed (2% to 4%).

INJECTION: Local corticosteroid injection is indicated for (1) recurrent nonseptic bursitis, (2) bursitis due to gout when NSAIDs are contraindicated, (3) chronic bursal thickening (palpably thickened soft tissues above the patella—the "bursal pinch sign"), or (4) persistent postinfectious bursitis (with a negative postantibiotic culture).

Positioning: The patient is placed in the supine position with the leg fully extended.
Surface Anatomy and the Point of Entry: The superior and inferior margins of the bursa are identified and marked. The point of entry is at the base of the inferior margin.
Angle of Entry and Depth: The needle is inserted at the base of the bursa, paralleling the patella, and advanced to the center of the bursa. Alternatively, the needle is entered above the bursa and advanced at a 45-degree angle down to the firm to hard resistance of the periosteum of the patella (for the chronically thickened bursa with little fluid).

Anesthesia: Ethyl chloride is sprayed on the skin. Local anesthetic is placed at the base of the bursa in the subcutaneous tissue and dermis only.
Technique: Complete aspiration of the contents of the bursa combined with bursal wall compression ensures the best outcome. After local anesthesia, an 18-gauge needle attached to a 10-mL syringe is passed into the center of the sac. The needle is rotated 180 degrees so that the

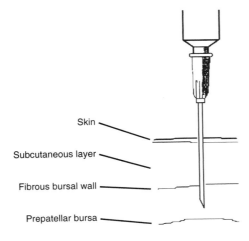

Skin

Subcutaneous layer

Fibrous bursal wall

Prepatellar bursa

Figure 9-7B Prepatellar bursa injection.

bevel faces the patella. Aspiration with gentle suction combined with manual pressure from above and the sides facilitates fluid removal. With the needle left in place, the syringe is replaced with the syringe containing the corticosteroid; 1 mL of K40 is injected. The needle is withdrawn and a gauze and Coban pressure dressing is applied.

INJECTION AFTERCARE

1. The knee must be *protected for the first 3 days* by avoiding direct pressure, all squatting, kneeling, and bending beyond 90 degrees.
2. The compression dressing is worn for 24 to 36 hours and then replaced with a neoprene pull-on knee sleeve.
3. *Ice* (15 minutes every 4 to 6 hours), *acetaminophen* (1000 mg twice a day), or both, are used for postinjection soreness.
4. The knee must be *protected* for 3 to 4 weeks by avoiding direct pressure (squatting and kneeling) and limiting bending to 90 degrees.
5. *Straight-leg-raise exercises* of the quadriceps muscle are begun on day 4 to recover any lost muscle tone.
6. *Aspiration and injection* with corticosteroid can be repeated at 6 weeks if swelling recurs or persists.
7. *Consultation* with a surgical orthopedist can be considered if two consecutive aspirations and injections fail to eliminate the swelling and pressure pain.

OUTCOME AND FURTHER WORK-UP: Ninety percent to 95% of patients with prepatellar bursitis respond to drainage and injection with corticosteroid. Patients with septic bursitis and those with persistent swelling that has been present for longer than 6 months have a greater risk of chronic bursitis (fibrosis, thickening, and recurrent effusion). Patients with signs of chronic bursitis are more likely to require bursectomy.

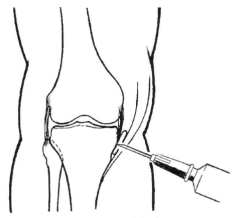

Enter at the point of maximum tenderness, usually 1½ inches below the medial joint line or parallel to the tibial tubercle in the concavity of the tibial plateau

Needle: 1- to 1½-inch, 22-gauge

Depth: ½ to 1½ inches exactly ⅛ inch above the periosteum of the tibia and outside the MCL

Volume: 1 to 2 mL anesthetic and 0.5 mL K40

NOTE: Never inject under forced pressure. The flow of medication should require little pressure when the injection is properly placed between the MCL and the conjoined tendon

Figure 9-8A   Anserine bursa injection.

SUMMARY

Anserine bursitis is an inflammation of the bursal sac located between the attachment of the MCL on the medial tibial plateau and the conjoined tendon formed by the gracilis, sartorius, and semitendinosus tendons. Although it can result from direct trauma, it more commonly develops as a result of an abnormal gait. Disruption of the normal mechanical relationship between the knee, hip, and pelvis causes an abnormal pull at the insertion point of the three tendons (the sartorius from the ileum, the gracilis from the pubis, and the semitendinosus from the ischium). The increased friction and pressure resulting from this gait disturbance cause anserine bursitis. It frequently accompanies osteoarthritis of the knee, chronic knee effusion, or any intrinsic knee condition.

TREATMENT OF CHOICE: When bursitis is the primary cause of knee pain, corticosteroid injection is the preferred initial treatment. When bursitis complicates one of the articular disorders of the knee or ankle, treatment must be directed at both.

SEQUENCE OF TREATMENTS

1. Treatment directed at the primary gait disturbance (knee effusion, osteoarthritis of the knee, leg length discrepancy, muscle imbalance from stroke) takes precedence when the symptoms arising from the primary condition outweigh the symptoms arising from the bursa.
2. *Injection:* Local anesthetic block is used to determine the contribution of the bursa to the patient's current symptoms.
3. Because the bursa lies superficially in most patients, ice over the anterior knee is a very effective analgesic.
4. *Acute restrictions:* Direct pressure must be avoided (including, placing a pillow between the knees while sleeping), and walking, standing, and repetitive bending must be limited.

5. ***Most common immobilizer:*** A pull-on neoprene sleeve can provide protection against direct pressure.
6. ***Injection:*** Local corticosteroid injection with depot methylprednisolone 80 mg/mL (D80) is appropriate for the patient with predominantly bursal symptoms.
7. ***Recovery exercise:*** Isometric straight-leg-raise exercises are performed to complete the recovery.

SURGICAL PROCEDURE: Rarely, bursectomy (1%).

INJECTION: Local injection is used to (1) to confirm the diagnosis, (2) treat primary bursitis, and (3) treat bursitis that persists after addressing the primary gait disturbance.

Positioning: The patient is placed in the supine position with the leg extended and externally rotated.

Surface Anatomy and the Point of Entry: The tibial tubercle, medial joint line, and the midline of the medial lower leg are identified and marked. The point of entry is in the midline directly across from the tibial tubercle or approximately $1\frac{1}{2}$ inches below the medial joint line.

Angle of Entry and Depth: The needle is inserted perpendicularly to the skin and is directed slightly upward toward the concavity of the medial tibial plateau. The injection depth is always $\frac{1}{8}$ inch above the periosteum of the tibia or $\frac{1}{2}$ to $1\frac{1}{2}$ inches deep.

Anesthesia: Ethyl chloride is sprayed on the skin. Local anesthetic is placed at the tissue plane of the tendon and $\frac{1}{8}$ inch above the periosteum of the tibia (both 0.5 mL).

Technique: A 22-gauge needle is passed through the subcutaneous fat until the subtle resistance of the conjoined tendon is felt. Anesthesia can be injected here for comfort. Then the needle is gently passed an additional $\frac{3}{8}$ inch to the firm periosteum of the tibia and immediately withdrawn $\frac{1}{8}$ inch to avoid injecting into the MCL. The bursa is located between the MCL and the tendon, and anesthetic and corticosteroid are injected here. Injection should be free flowing with little resistance. Pressure on injection usually suggests improper position (too deep!).

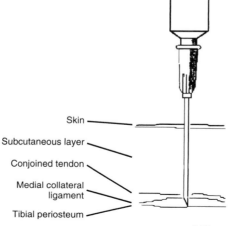

Skin

Subcutaneous layer

Conjoined tendon

Medial collateral ligament

Tibial periosteum

Figure 9-8B Anserine bursa injection.

140

INJECTION AFTERCARE

1. The knee must be *protected for the first 3 days* by avoiding direct pressure, all squatting, kneeling, and bending beyond 90 degrees.
2. Crutches with touch-down weightbearing for 3 to 7 days are necessary only if the underlying gait disturbance is severe.
3. *Ice* (15 minutes every 4 to 6 hours), *acetaminophen* (1000 mg twice a day), or both, are used for postinjection soreness.
4. The knee must be *protected* for 3 to 4 weeks by limiting direct pressure and repetitive bending, and unnecessary walking.
5. *Straight-leg-raise exercises* of the quadriceps muscle are begun on day 4 to enhance support of the knee.
6. For those patients with poor quadriceps muscle tone or with frequent giving out of the knee, temporary bracing (3 to 4 weeks) with a patellar restraining brace or a Velcro straight leg is recommended.
7. *Injection* can be repeated at 6 weeks with corticosteroid if pain and swelling persist.
8. If the initial treatment response is unsatisfactory, *plain film radiographs* (standing PA knees, bilateral sunrise views) or *MRI* is obtained to identify advanced degenerative arthritis, high degree subluxation of the patellofemoral joint, degenerative or traumatic meniscal tear, and so forth.
9. Long-term restrictions of bending (30 to 45 degrees) and the impact of weightbearing are advised for the patient with chronic symptoms.
10. *Consultation* with an orthopedist is indicated for the management of the underlying gait disturbance

OUTCOME AND FURTHER WORK-UP: Primary involvement of the bursa and secondary anserine bursitis—associated with an underlying gait disturbance—respond dramatically to corticosteroid injection. Primary bursitis responds dramatically and completely to injection. Further work-up is not necessary in these cases. However, the injection response may be short lived with secondary bursitis if the underlying knee effusion, arthritis, short leg, or other gait disturbance is not treated concurrently. Any patient with persistent anserine bursitis must undergo a thorough evaluation of the gait, knee, hip, and ankle, both by examination and radiographically.

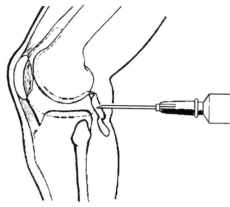

Enter over the center of the cyst with
the needle held vertically
Needle: 1½-inch, 18-gauge
Depth: ¾ to 1¼ inches
Volume: 1 to 2 mL anesthetic and
1 mL K40
NOTE: The cyst is located in the fatty
layer! The neurovascular bundle is
deep to the cyst. Use continuous
light vacuum pressure while
advancing the needle

Figure 9-9A   Baker's cyst aspiration and injection.

SUMMARY

A Baker's cyst is an abnormal collection of synovial fluid in the fatty layers of the popliteal fossa. It must be distinguished from the much more common dilated semimembranosus bursa—an evagination of the synovial lining of the knee—which gradually enlarges as a result of the hydraulic pressure of repetitive flexing of the knee. Both are located on the medial side of the popliteal fossa and both result from an overproduction of synovial fluid. However, only the Baker's cyst is a separate anatomic structure. Small cysts should be observed. Large Baker's cysts that interfere with flexion of the knee can be aspirated and injected with corticosteroids. Dilated semimembranosus bursae are not aspirated and injected directly. The treatment for a dilated bursa is directed at the underlying cause (osteoarthritis, rheumatoid arthritis, meniscal tear, etc.).

TREATMENT OF CHOICE: Whether the cyst is a Baker's cyst or simply a dilated bursa, few need to be treated directly. In general, treatment should be directed at the primary knee condition causing the overproduction of fluid. However, if the cyst is large or if it interferes with full flexion of the knee or if the patient insists on treatment, local aspiration and corticosteroid injection of the cyst can be considered.

SEQUENCE OF TREATMENTS

1. Attention should be paid to treating the underlying cause of the knee effusion such as osteoarthritis, rheumatoid arthritis, and so forth.
2. *Injection:* Aspiration is used to confirm the diagnosis (typical high viscosity fluid) and corticosteroid injection with K40 is used to treat the large cysts that interfere with full knee flexion (see details on page 143).
3. *Acute restrictions:* Walking and standing should be limited and repetitive bending (flexion limited to 30 to 45 degrees) should be avoided.
4. *Exercise of choice:* As for most knee conditions, isometric straight-leg-raises are recommended.

5. ***Most common immobilizer:*** No specific brace is used for popliteal cysts; a pull-on neoprene knee sleeve provides warmth and nominal support.
6. ***Consultation:*** Orthopedic consultation can be considered for cysts that repeatedly accumulate large amounts of fluid and that interfere with full flexion.
7. ***Recovery exercises:*** The straight-leg-raise exercise combined with hamstring leg extensions completes the recovery.

SURGICAL PROCEDURE: Occasionally, bursectomy.

INJECTION: Aspiration is used to confirm the diagnosis (typical high-viscosity fluid), and corticosteroid injection with K40 is used to treat the large cysts that interfere with full knee flexion.

Positioning: The patient is placed in the prone position with the leg fully extended.

Surface Anatomy and the Point of Entry: The outline of the cyst is marked, typically an oblong structure located medially in the popliteal fossa and extending inferiorly. The point of entry is directly over the center of the cyst.

Angle of Entry and Depth: The needle is inserted perpendicular to the skin and is advanced through the subcutaneous tissue to the subtle tissue resistance of the cyst wall ($\frac{3}{4}$ to $1\frac{1}{4}$ inches below the skin surface).

Anesthesia: Ethyl chloride is sprayed on the skin. Using a 22-gauge needle, local anesthetic is placed intradermally, subcutaneously, and just outside the cyst wall (0.5 mL).

Technique: An 18-gauge needle attached to a 20-mL syringe is held vertically and passed down to the subtle resistance of the cyst wall. Note that the neurovascular bundle is deep to the cyst; only skin and subcutaneous overly the cyst cavity! Continuous negative pressure is used while advancing. The outer wall is often quite thick and a giving way or popping sensation is often felt

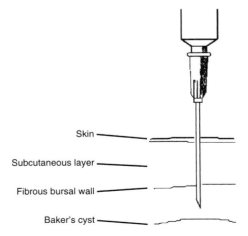

Skin

Subcutaneous layer

Fibrous bursal wall

Baker's cyst

Figure 9-9B   Baker's cyst injection.

as the cyst is entered. After the cyst is punctured, the syringe is removed, and the needle is gently advanced until the subtle tissue resistance of the back wall is felt or fluid can no longer be easily aspirated. At this point the needle is withdrawn $\frac{1}{8}$ to $\frac{3}{8}$ inch. This needle position will ensure optimal aspiration of the fluid as the cyst collapses. Manual pressure is applied to either side of the needle to assist in fluid recovery. With the needle left in place, 1 mL of K40 is injected into the cyst.

INJECTION AFTERCARE
1. The knee must be ***protected for the first 3 days*** by avoiding direct pressure, squatting, kneeling, and bending beyond 90 degrees.
2. Crutches with touch-down weightbearing for 3 to 7 days are necessary only if the underlying condition affecting the knee is severe.
3. ***Ice*** (15 minutes every 4 to 6 hours), ***acetaminophen*** (1000 mg twice a day), or both, are used for postinjection soreness.
4. The knee must be ***protected*** for 3 to 4 weeks by limiting direct pressure, bending, squatting, kneeling, impact, and unnecessary walking.
5. ***Straight-leg-raise exercises*** of the quadriceps muscle are begun on day 4 to enhance support of the knee.
6. Maximize the treatment of the associated condition affecting the knee (osteoarthritis, rheumatoid arthritis, etc.).
7. ***Aspiration and injection*** can be repeated at 6 weeks if pain recurs or persists.
8. ***Consultation*** with a surgical orthopedist can be considered if two consecutive aspirations and injections fail to eliminate the swelling and the patient still complains of pressure and swelling in the popliteal fossa.

OUTCOME AND FURTHER WORK-UP: In the short term, the optimal treatment of a Baker's cyst depends on the complete aspiration of its contents and the accurate placement of the corticosteroid. However, the long-term prognosis is always dependent on the underlying process affecting the knee. Work-up and treatment are always directed to evaluating and controlling the associated knee effusion.

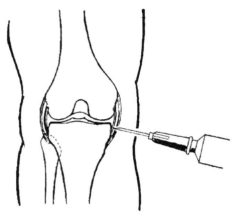

Enter in the midline over the tibial plateau just below the joint line
Needle: $^5/_8$-inch, 25-gauge or $1^1/_2$-inch, 22-gauge
Depth: Varies according to the thickness of the dermis, averaging $^1/_2$ to $^3/_4$ inch; alternatively, $^1/_8$ inch above the periosteum of the tibia
Volume: 1 to 2 mL anesthetic and 1 mL K40
NOTE: Never inject between the MCL and the bone; and always brace after injection

Figure 9-10A   Medial collateral ligament (MCL) injection.

SUMMARY

A MCL sprain is an injury of the inner "hinge" ligament of the knee. Sprains are classified as first, second, or third degree on the basis of the amount of motion on valgus stress testing. Dramatic twisting of the knee or falls that place the knee in a valgus position are the types of injuries that are common to all degrees of sprain. Ligaments that are irritated and inflamed but otherwise intact are classified as first-degree sprains. Ligaments that are partially torn are classified as second-degree separations. Ligaments that are completely disrupted with gross instability of the knee are classified as third-degree separations. Patients with third-degree separations must be evaluated for coexisting injuries to the ACL, medial meniscus, or both.

TREATMENT OF CHOICE: Immobilization with a Velcro straight-leg immobilizer or a patellar restraining brace is combined with crutches and physical therapy exercises.

SEQUENCE OF TREATMENTS

1. *Most common immobilizer:* A Velcro straight-leg immobilizer is preferred for higher-grade injuries and is combined with crutches for 7 to 14 days.
2. *Acute restrictions:* Bending, twisting, and pivoting must be avoided and in higher-grade injuries can be combined with crutches for 7 to 14 days.
3. Ice placed over the medial joint line is an effective analgesic.
4. *Exercise of choice:* Isometric straight-leg-raise exercises are performed daily initially in the knee brace with a gradually transition out of the brace.
5. *Injection:* Local corticosteroid injection with D80 can be used if symptoms and signs fail to improve between 4 and 6 weeks (see details on page 146).
6. *Recovery exercises:* Isometric straight-leg-raise exercises and hamstring extensions are used to recover full muscular support to the knee.

7. *Consultation:* Orthopedic consultation is strongly recommended for third-degree sprains with associated injuries and for lesser sprains that have failed to improve after 2 to 3 months.

SURGICAL PROCEDURE: The decision to proceed with surgery with the higher-grade ligament injuries must be made early. A choice between primary repair or delayed reconstruction for third-degree tears is based on the degree of instability and the coexistent injuries.

INJECTION: Immobilization combined with physical therapy strengthening exercises are the treatments of choice. The use of local corticosteroid injection is adjunctive at best and is appropriate only for first and second degree that fails to improve with immobilization, the quadriceps toning exercise, and several weeks of restricted use.

Position: The patient is placed in the supine position with the leg extended and externally rotated.

Surface Anatomy and the Point of Entry: The MCL is located in the midplane originating at the medial femoral condyle and inserting on the medial tibial plateau. The point of entry is just below the medial joint line on the tibia (the joint line is located parallel to the lower third of the patella when the leg is in the extended position).

Angle of Entry and Depth: The needle is inserted in the midplane on the tibial side of the medial joint line perpendicular to the skin. The depth is $\frac{1}{8}$ inch above the periosteum of the tibia, approximately $\frac{1}{2}$ to $\frac{3}{4}$ inch from the skin.

Anesthesia: Ethyl chloride is sprayed on the skin. Local anesthetic is placed subcutaneously and $\frac{1}{8}$ inch above the tibial periosteum (0.5 mL).

Technique: The tibial plateau is identified, just below the medial joint line. A 25-gauge needle is inserted, held perpendicular to the skin, and advanced down to the firm resistance of the periosteum of the tibia. Once the bone has been encountered, the needle is withdrawn $\frac{1}{8}$ inch to ensure the injection is above the MCL attachment (error on the superficial side rather than too deep; deep injections may detach a portion of the ligament off the bone). Do not inject if firm or

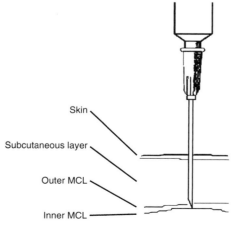

Skin

Subcutaneous layer

Outer MCL

Inner MCL

Figure 9-10B Medial collateral ligament (MCL) injection.

hard pressure is encountered (too deep)! After local anesthesia, reassess tenderness and pain and movement with valgus stress testing. If these signs are significantly improved with less pain, inject the same area with 0.5 mL of D80. Massage the medication in for 1 to 2 minutes.

INJECTION AFTERCARE

1. The knee must be *protected for the first 3 days* by avoiding direct pressure, all twisting, squatting, kneeling, and repetitive bending.
2. Crutches with touch-down weightbearing are strongly suggested for the first 3 to 7 days.
3. The Velcro straight-leg immobilizer should be worn continuously during the day for mild to moderate injuries and 24 hours for severe injuries.
4. *Ice* (15 minutes every 4 to 6 hours), *acetaminophen* (1000 mg twice a day), or both, are used for postinjection soreness.
5. The knee must be *protected* for 3 to 4 weeks by limiting direct pressure, repetitive bending, and unnecessary walking; the knee immobilizer should be worn during the day.
6. *Straight-leg-raise exercises* of the quadriceps muscle are begun on day 4 to enhance support of the knee (perform these in the brace for the first week or two).
7. *Injection* with corticosteroid can be repeated at 6 weeks if pain recurs or persists.
8. Request a *consultation* with a surgical orthopedist if two consecutive injections fail and the patient still complains of pain with pivoting and twisting (internal derangement?).

OUTCOME AND FURTHER WORK-UP: Most MCL sprains occur as a result of trauma. The sprain is either an isolated process (minor twisting injuries or simple falls; better prognosis) or associated with tears to the meniscal cartilage or anterior cruciate ligament (major trauma; guarded prognosis). MCL injury may also develop as a complication of an underlying effusion or arthritis. The ligament has a greater vulnerability to injury in the presence of a large chronic effusions (stretching of the supporting structures) and the arthritic narrowing of the medial cartilage (laxity of the ligament due to narrowing of the joint). In either case, depending on the severity of the injury, MRI, arthroscopy, or both are necessary to define the extent of the injury. Immobilization, physical therapy, and rest remain the mainstays of early treatment for first- and second-degree sprains and surgical intervention for third-degree sprains. Ultimately, the outcome depends on the degree of injury, associated injuries, and underlying knee pathology.

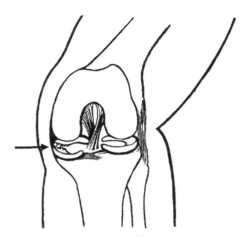

Tears are classified by size as partial or complete; by location as anterior, lateral or posterior; by cause as traumatic or degenerative; or by description as horizontal, vertical, radial, parrot beak or bucket handle

Figure 9-11   Medial meniscal tear.

SUMMARY

A torn meniscus is a disruption of the unique fibrocartilage pad located between the femoral condyle and the tibial plateau. Tears are classified as partial or complete, anterior, lateral or posterior, traumatic or degenerative, or horizontal, vertical, radial, parrot beak, or bucket handle. Because of the strategic location and inherent shock-absorbing properties of the meniscus, meniscal tears lead to a loss of smooth motion of the knee, variable degrees of the classic locking phenomenon, loss of full extension of the knee, and knee effusions. Patients suspected of having a torn meniscus must undergo either MRI or arthroscopy to confirm the diagnosis. Small tears that do not extend to the articular cartilage of the femur or tibia can be observed; these have the least potential for further joint damage. Moderate to large tears that extend to the articular cartilage are more significant, tend to cause greater degrees of knee swelling and loss of normal mechanical function of the knee, and as such, are more likely to require surgery.

TREATMENT OF CHOICE: Arthroscopy is used to confirm the diagnosis and inspect the articular surfaces for associated injury. Meniscectomy is the treatment of choice for the large, complex tears that have potential for continued damage to cartilage.

SEQUENCE OF TREATMENTS

1.   Athletic activities must be interrupted to avoid further injury to the knee.
2.   *Most common immobilizer:* A patellar restraining brace for general support can be combined with crutches, depending on the severity of the injury.
3.   *Restrictions:* All twisting and pivoting must be absolutely avoided and impact and repetitive bending need to be limited.
4.   *Exercise of choice:* Initially the isometric straight-leg-raise exercise is performed in the brace and with improvement without the brace.

148

5. ***Injection:*** An intra-articular injection of local anesthesia is occasionally used to distinguish the presence of an intra-articular process (optional).
6. Aspiration and drainage of "tense" hemorrhagic effusions reduces pain, allows greater involvement in recovery exercises, and decreases the chance of further cartilage damage.
7. Many small meniscal tears that are unassociated with persistent effusion and mechanical dysfunction will gradually or spontaneous resolve over time, arguing for a period of observation over several months.
8. ***Consultation:*** Arthroscopy is the procedure of choice to define the extent of the problem and determine the need for definitive meniscectomy.
9. ***Recovery exercises:*** Straight-leg-raise exercises combined with hamstring leg extensions complete the recovery.

SURGICAL PROCEDURE: Partial meniscectomy is the preferred surgical procedure because it attempts to preserve as much of the normal shock-absorbing properties of the meniscus as possible.

INJECTION: For large meniscal tears that interfere with the normal, smooth motion of the knee, arthroscopy with débridement is the treatment of choice. However, aspiration of the knee can be used as an interim treatment and is recommended to rapidly reduce the pressure symptoms of the acute, tense bloody effusion. In addition, local corticosteroid injection is recommended in the select group of patients with osteoarthritis complicated by a degenerative meniscal tear (see the technique of knee aspiration on pages 129-130).

OUTCOME AND FURTHER WORK-UP: Meniscal tear is a classic mechanical problem affecting the knee. Surgical evaluation and treatment rather than anti-inflammatory treatments is relied upon to restore the normal function of the knee. Unless the meniscal tear occurs in the setting of a primary arthritis (with a component of active inflammation), corticosteroid injection provides minimal relief. Furthermore, short-lived response (days) to a properly placed intra-articular corticosteroid often suggests mechanical issues are the dominant process. Patients with poor responses to corticosteroid injection should be evaluated by MRI, arthroscopy, or both to define the extent of the process.

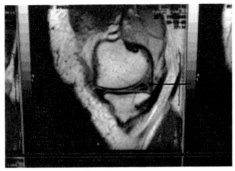

Figure 9-12   Magnetic resonance imaging (MRI), Lateral View, Demonstrating a Horizontal Tear *(arrow)*—This is an example of a horizontal tear of the medial meniscus, extending to the surface of the articular cartilage of the tibia. This type of tear interferes with the normal function of the knee and poses a threat to the tibial cartilage. Clinically, the patient complained of a loss of smooth motion, a sense of catching, and intermittent anterior swelling. Tears that extend to the surface of the articular cartilage and multidirectional complex tears have the potential to cause symptoms, cause injury to articular cartilage, and accelerate osteoarthritis. Contrast this with the common radiographic finding "mucinoid degenerative change," an age-related defect located centrally in the meniscus. This incidental finding does not extend to the articular surface and as such does not cause symptoms and pose a risk to accelerated wear-and-tear. These differences between meniscal lesions underscore the need to be cautions when interpreting MRI. Imaging is indicated for the following: patients who have suffered injury; patients with classic mechanical symptoms such as ratcheting, locking, and so forth; young athletic patients with an unexplained knee effusion but normal plain films; patients with acute hemarthrosis; and patients with osteoarthritis who have suffered an injury and a dramatic increase in knee symptoms.

Chapter 10

ANKLE AND LOWER LEG

THE DIFFERENTIAL DIAGNOSIS OF ANKLE AND LOWER LEG PAIN

DIAGNOSES	CONFIRMATIONS
Ligaments (most common)	
Ankle sprain (first, second, third degree)	Examination; radiographs (if indicated)
Ankle sprain with fibular avulsion	Examination; radiographs (ankle series)
Ankle sprain with peroneus tendon avulsion fracture	Examination; radiographs (ankle series)
Ankle sprain with osteochondritis dissecans or chondral fracture	Examination; radiographs; magnetic resonance imaging (MRI)
Ankle sprain with interosseus membrane disruption	Examination; radiographs (stress views)
Ankle sprain with instability	Examination; radiographs (stress views)
Tendons	
Achilles tendinitis	Examination; MRI
Achilles tendon rupture	Examination; MRI
Peroneus tenosynovitis	Local anesthetic block
Posterior tibialis tenosynovitis	Local anesthetic block
Bursa	
Pre-Achilles bursitis	Local anesthetic block
Retrocalcaneal bursitis	Local anesthetic block
Joint	
Osteoarthritis, post-traumatic	Radiographs: ankle series
Inflammatory or septic arthritis	Aspiration/synovial fluid analysis
Heel	
Heel pad syndrome	Examination
Plantar fasciitis	Local anesthetic block
Sever's disease (age younger than 18 years)	Radiographs: ankle series
Calcaneal stress fracture	Radiographs or bone scanning
Tarsal tunnel syndrome	Nerve conduction velocity testing
Referred pain	
Lumbosacral spine radiculopathy	Computed tomography (CT) scan; MRI; electromyogram
Compartment syndrome/shinsplints	Calf examination
Baker's cyst	Knee examination; ultrasound

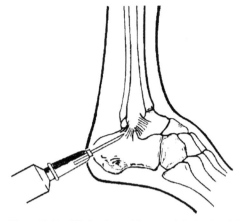

Enter $\frac{1}{2}$ inch anterior to the lateral
malleolus for the talofibular
ligament and $\frac{1}{2}$ inch below the tip
of the lateral malleolus for the
fibulocalcaneal ligament
Needle: $\frac{5}{8}$-inch, 25-gauge
Depth: $\frac{1}{2}$ to $\frac{5}{8}$ inch
Volume: 1 to 2 mL anesthetic and
0.5 mL D80
NOTE: Confirm the placement with
local anesthetic first; immobilize for
1 to 4 weeks after corticosteroid
injection, depending on the severity

Figure 10-1A   Fibulocalcaneal ligament injection just below the inferior tip of the lateral malleolus.

SUMMARY

An ankle sprain is a partial tear of the supporting ligaments of the ankle joint. Inversion injuries cause the fibulocalcaneal or the fibulotalar ligaments to microsplit, microtear, or microavulse from their normal bony attachments. Sprains are classified as acute, recurrent, or chronic. Ligaments that do not heal properly and do not reattach to their bony origins can cause significant ankle instability, which, in turn, can lead to recurrent ankle sprain, osteoarthritis, or osteochondritis dissecans.

TREATMENT OF CHOICE: Immobilization of the ankle, lower leg, or both is the treatment of choice, including high-top shoes, overlap-taping, an air cast, or a short-leg walking cast.

SEQUENCE OF TREATMENTS

1. Ice and elevation are effective in reducing swelling and pain.
2. *Most common immobilizers:* For mild sprains, immobilization with high-top shoes or overlap-taping for 2 to 3 weeks is sufficient; severe sprains require 3 to 4 weeks of protection in an air cast or a short-leg walking cast.
3. Crutches using touch-down weightbearing are optional in the first week.
4. *Acute restrictions:* Walking, standing, impact, and repetitive bending should be avoided.
5. *Exercises of choice:* Although controversial, this author prefers to begin passive range of motion exercises to restore full ankle flexibility after a period of strict immobilization.
6. *Recovery exercises:* After the pain and swelling have dissipated, isometric toning exercises of eversion are begun to provide additional support laterally.
7. *Injection:* Local anesthetic block may be necessary to distinguish involvement of the joint and peroneus tendons from injury to the supporting ligaments; corticosteroid injection with depot

methylprednisolone 80 mg/mL (D80) has limited indications—only if inflammation, swelling, and pain persist despite immobilization and physical therapy (see details on page 153).

8. ***Consultation:*** Orthopedic consultation is indicated when pain and instability persist.
9. Gradual return to athletic and sports activities completes the rehabilitation process.

SURGICAL PROCEDURE: Advanced third-degree tears can be repaired primarily or undergo delayed reconstruction if the ankle remains unstable.

INJECTION: Immobilization combined with physical therapy strengthening exercises is the treatment of choice. Local corticosteroid injection is not commonly performed and is reserved for first-degree sprains that remain inflamed, painful, and swollen.

Position: The patient is placed in the supine position. The ankle is kept in neutral position.
Surface Anatomy and the Point of Entry: The tip of the lateral malleolus and the point of maximum tenderness are identified and marked. The point of entry is $\frac{1}{2}$ inch anterior or $\frac{1}{2}$ inch inferior to the lateral malleolus (depending on which ligament has been injured, the fibulotalar and fibulocalcaneal ligaments, respectively).
Angle of Entry and Depth: The needle is inserted directly over the point of maximum tenderness, perpendicular to the skin. The depth is $\frac{1}{2}$ to $\frac{5}{8}$ inch from the skin.

Anesthesia: Ethyl chloride is sprayed on the skin. Local anesthetic is placed subcutaneously and at the firm resistance of the lateral ligament $\frac{1}{4}$ to $\frac{1}{2}$ inch from the skin (0.5 mL).
Technique: All medication injections should be placed atop the ligament—between the subcutaneous tissue and the ligament. This tissue plane can be easily identified by advancing the needle gradually until the firm resistance of the ligament is appreciated or until the tip of the needle sticks in place when skin traction is applied (if the needle is above the ligament, the needle will move with the skin and subcutaneous tissue when traction is applied). After local anesthesia,

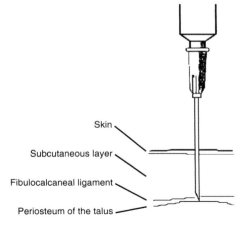

Skin

Subcutaneous layer

Fibulocalcaneal ligament

Periosteum of the talus

Figure 10-1B Fibulocalcaneal ligament injection.

the ankle is reexamined for instability and pain relief. If local tenderness and passive inversion are no longer as painful and the ankle shows no sign of gross instability (the anterior drawer and talar knock signs are negative), 0.5 mL of D80 is injected.

INJECTION AFTERCARE

1. The ankle must be *protected for the first 3 days* by avoiding all unnecessary weightbearing (it takes 3 days for the medication to set up).
2. Crutches with touch-down weightbearing are strongly suggested for the first 3 to 7 days.
3. Immobilization with lace-up high-top shoes, an air cast, or a short-leg walking cast for 1 to 4 weeks is used, depending on the severity of the injury.
4. *Ice* (15 minutes every 4 to 6 hours), *acetaminophen (Tylenol ES)* (1000 mg twice a day), or both, are used for postinjection soreness.
5. Movement of the ankle must be *restricted* for 3 to 4 weeks by avoiding all twisting and pivoting and limiting unnecessary walking and standing.
6. *Isometric toning exercises* of ankle eversion and inversion are begun at 3 to 4 weeks to enhance ankle support.
7. *Injection* with corticosteroid can be repeated at 6 weeks if pain persists.
8. *Consultation* with a surgical orthopedist can be considered if immobilization, physical therapy, and two consecutive injections fail and the patient still complains of pain with pivoting and twisting (internal derangement?).

OUTCOME AND FURTHER WORK-UP: Most sprained ankles respond to rest and immobilization. For severe ankle sprains (unable to bear weight, goose-egg-sized swelling, intolerance of passive range of motion testing in inversion, and bony tenderness), error on the side of immobilization. The best outcome can be achieved by combining immobilization with various other treatments (1) that maximize the anatomic reattachment of the ligament, (2) minimize future recurrent ankle sprains, and (3) avoid ankle joint instability. Persistent pain and swelling suggest poor healing of the original ligament injury or possible unrecognized injury to the adjacent bones, tendons, or ankle cartilage. Patients who fail to resolve their injury in 4 to 6 weeks should undergo stress views of the ankle for instability, MRI for osteochondritis dissecans, nuclear medicine bone scanning for occult bony fracture, or synovial fluid analysis for injury to the ankle or subtalar joint.

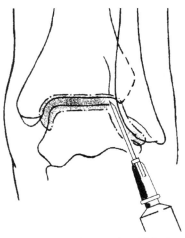

The ankle can be entered anteromedially just medial to the extensor hallucis longus or anterolaterally just lateral to the extensor digiti minimi

Needle: 1½-inch, 22-gauge

Depth: 1 to 1¼ inches through either the tibionavicular ligament medially or the tibionavicular ligament laterally

Volume: 2 to 3 mL anesthetic and 0.5 mL K40

NOTE: If bone is encountered, withdraw back through the ligament, use skin traction to redirect the needle either toward the midline or inferiorly, and advance again

Figure 10-2A Arthrocentesis and injection of the ankle.

SUMMARY

Effusion of the ankle is an uncommon problem. Swelling at the ankle is more often due to edema (fluid retention, congestive heart failure, varicosities, deep venous thrombosis), ankle sprain, or fracture. True ankle effusion presents as a bandlike swelling that forms over the anterior ankle joint, obliterates the malleolar prominences, and impairs dorsi- and plantar flexion of the joint. Aspiration and synovial fluid analysis of the tibiotalar joint are necessary to differentiate among the variety of causes of ankle effusion. These include traumatic bloody effusions, noninflammatory effusions due to osteoarthritis, inflammatory effusions due to rheumatoid disease, and the rare case of septic arthritis.

TREATMENT OF CHOICE: Ice, elevation, and limited weightbearing are always indicated. However, a definitive diagnosis requires aspiration and diagnostic studies, providing the practitioner with the best guidelines for therapy.

SEQUENCE OF TREATMENTS

1. Diagnostic aspiration is used to differentiate inflammatory arthritis and septic arthritis from hemarthrosis (see synovial fluid analysis table, page 210).
2. Ice and elevation are effective in reducing pain and swelling.
3. *Most common immobilizers:* The joint can be protected by immobilization with high-top shoes (mild disease), Velcro ankle brace, or an air cast (moderate disease), or with a walking cast combined with touch-down weightbearing with crutches (severe disease).
4. *Restrictions:* Walking, standing, impact, and repetitive bending must be restricted until the swelling and pain are well controlled.

5. A 2- to 3-week trial of a nonsteroidal anti-inflammatory drug (NSAID) is effective for mild involvement.
6. *Injection:* Local corticosteroid injection with triamcinolone acetonide 40 mg/mL (K40) provides the most predictable outcome for the nonseptic effusion (see below).
7. *Recovery exercises:* Passive range of motion exercises are used to restore full ankle flexibility and are typically performed after 3 weeks of fixed immobilization. Subsequently, isometric toning exercises of eversion and inversion are performed daily to enhance ankle support.
8. *Consultation:* Orthopedic consultation can be considered for advanced disease associated with greater than 50% loss of range of motion and intractable pain.

SURGICAL PROCEDURE: Patients with moderate involvement can be considered for arthroscopic débridement, particularly those with loose bodies, osteochondritis dissecans, and advanced arthritis. Patients with advanced wear-and-tear of the joint, intractable pain, and poor function are candidates for arthrodesis.

INJECTION: Ice, elevation, and limited weightbearing are always indicated for significant ankle effusion. Diagnostic aspiration is mandatory if septic arthritis is suspected. Local corticosteroid injection is indicated for large or persistent nonseptic effusions.

Position: The patient is placed in the supine position and the ankle is held in 15 to 20 degrees of plantar flexion (this tightens the anterior capsule).

Surface Anatomy and the Point of Entry: A horizontal line is drawn $\frac{1}{2}$ inch above the tip of the medial malleolus and $\frac{3}{4}$ inch above the tip of the lateral malleolus. The point of entry is at the intersection of these lines and just lateral to the extensor digiti minimi **(anterolateral approach)** or, alternatively, just medial to the extensor hallucis longus **(anteromedially).**

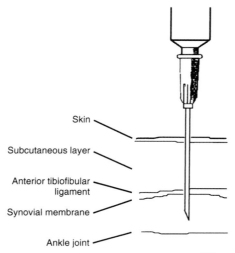

Skin

Subcutaneous layer

Anterior tibiofibular ligament

Synovial membrane

Ankle joint

Figure 10-2B Ankle joint injection.

Angle of Entry and Depth: The needle is inserted perpendicular to the skin and angled toward the center of the joint. The depth is 1 to $1\frac{1}{4}$ inches from the skin.

Anesthesia: Ethyl chloride is sprayed on the skin. Local anesthetic is placed subcutaneously, at the firm resistance of the extensor retinaculum, and intra-articularly (0.5 mL).

Technique: The **anterolateral approach** is preferred because the extent of the lateral synovial cavity is greater and there are fewer obstructing structures to encounter. Following the placement of anesthetic in the superficial dermis, the 22-gauge needle is slowly advanced through the firm resistance of the extensor retinaculum and superficial ligaments. If bone is encountered at $\frac{1}{2}$ inch (tibia, talus, or fibula), the needle must be withdrawn through the superficial tissues, repositioned with the aid of skin traction either up or down or medially. If the needle is centered over the joint, the passage of the needle to a depth of 1 to $1\frac{1}{4}$ inches should be smooth and unobstructed. Note that the joint cannot be entered if the needle is more than 15 to 20 degrees from perpendicular. If active infection is excluded by fluid inspection or subsequent synovial fluid laboratory analysis, 0.5 mL K40 is injected intra-articularly.

INJECTION AFTERCARE

1. The ankle must be ***protected for the first 3 days*** by avoiding all unnecessary weightbearing (it takes 3 days for the medication to set up).
2. Crutches with touch-down weightbearing are strongly suggested for the first 3 to 7 days.
3. Immobilization with lace-up high-top shoes, an air cast, or a short-leg walking cast is recommended for 1 to 4 weeks, depending on the severity of the arthritis and swelling.
4. ***Ice*** (15 minutes every 4 to 6 hours), ***acetaminophen*** (1000 mg twice a day), or both, are used for postinjection soreness.
5. Movement of the ankle must be ***restricted*** for 3 to 4 weeks by avoiding all twisting and pivoting and limiting unnecessary walking and standing.
6. ***Passive stretching exercises*** of the ankle in flexion and extension are begun after the pain and swelling have significantly improved.
7. ***Isometric toning exercises*** of ankle eversion and inversion to enhance the support of the ankle (always maintaining the ankle in neutral position) are begun at 3 to 4 weeks.
8. ***Injection*** with corticosteroid can be repeated at 6 weeks if pain and swelling persist.
9. Request an MRI and a ***consultation*** with a surgical orthopedist if two consecutive injections fail and the patient still complains of weightbearing pain (loose bodies, osteochondritis dissecans of the talar dome, etc.).

OUTCOME AND FURTHER WORK-UP: To ensure optimal results, corticosteroid injection should be combined with fixed immobilization. Work-up should always include synovial fluid analysis in order to differentiate rheumatoid, osteoarthritic, and crystal-induced arthritis from the very uncommon septic arthritis. If only a small amount of fluid is obtained, laboratory testing is prioritized to Gram stain and culture, and, if enough fluid is obtained, cell count and differential. MRI and bone scanning are used in the elusive case. These are used to evaluate the integrity of the articular cartilage (osteochondritis dissecans and chondral fracture) and the adjacent bones (bony cysts, occult fracture, avascular necrosis, and so forth).

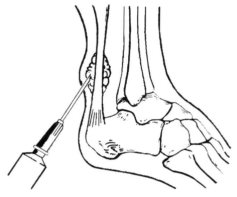

This is a peritendinous injection; enter along the outer edge of the tendon, approximately 1½ inches above the calcaneus
Needle: 1½-inch, 22-gauge
Depth: superficial—⅜ to ½ inch
Volume: 2 to 3 mL anesthetic and 1 mL D80, 0.5 mL injected on either side of the tendon
NOTE: Do not enter the tendon; minimal pressure is needed when injecting; immobilize with an air cast or short-leg walking cast for 3 to 4 weeks

Figure 10-3A   Peritendinous injection for Achilles tendinitis.

SUMMARY

Achilles tendinitis is an inflammation of the musculotendinous junction (MTJ) of the Achilles tendon, located approximately 1½ inches above the calcaneal insertion. Repetitive jumping, pivoting, and impact at the ankle causes inflammation in and around the tendon, mucinoid degenerative change, microtearing, and eventually peritendinous thickening. These pathologic changes weaken the tendon and can lead to complete tendon rupture in up to 10% of cases. Runners; patients with short, tight Achilles tendons; and patients with Reiter's disease are at particular risk for tendon rupture. Dramatic changes in the level of activity, incomplete warm-ups before sports, and inadequate stretching of the tendons predispose to tendinitis and rupture.

TREATMENT OF CHOICE: For Achilles tendinitis unassociated with tear, immobilization either with an air cast or a short-leg walking cast is the treatment of choice.

SEQUENCE OF TREATMENTS

1. Mildly symptomatic Achilles tendinitis can be treated with ice, restricted use, gradual tendon stretching, and measures to reduce friction over the tendon (double socks, mole foam, New-Skin, or adhesive pads).
2. ***Most common immobilizer:*** Moderate to severe cases should be treated with fixed immobilization for 3 to 4 weeks (air cast or a short-leg walking cast).
3. ***Recovery exercise:*** If symptoms are improved with immobilization, passive Achilles tendon stretches are begun.
4. ***Injection:*** If immobilization fails to control symptoms, the health care provider must choose between MRI to rule out a torn tendon or corticosteroid injection with D80 to treat persistent tendinitis (see details on page 159).
5. ***Consultation:*** Surgical consultation is indicated for refractory symptoms, especially if there is any indication of tear.
6. Isometric toning exercises are begun if active tendinitis has been controlled and once flexibility has been significantly improved (comparable to the unaffected side).

7. All activities must be restricted until all signs of irritation have resolved, full flexibility has been restored, and strength has been recovered.

SURGICAL PROCEDURE: Operative intervention for chronic Achilles tendinitis involves close inspection for subtle tendon tears followed by stripping away the peritendinous fibrosis. Primary repair of the tendon is the procedure of choice when the tendon has been torn.

INJECTION: The role of local injection remains controversial. Local corticosteroid injection can effectively reduce the chronic peritendinous inflammation and thickening. However, benefits of injection must be balanced against the risk of tendon rupture. To minimize this risk, it is strongly advised to combine injection with rigid immobilization.

Position: The patient is placed in the prone position with the foot hanging over the end of the examination table. The ankle is kept in a neutral position.

Surface Anatomy and the Point of Entry: The peritendinous thickening surrounding the tendon is identified. The two points of entry are on either side of the thickening.

Angle of Entry and Depth: The needle is inserted along side the tendon at the level of the peritendinous thickening, at an angle paralleling the tendon. The depth is $\frac{3}{8}$ to $\frac{1}{2}$ inch from the surface.

Anesthesia: Ethyl chloride is sprayed on the skin. Local anesthetic is placed subcutaneously (0.5 mL) and adjacent to the peritendinous thickening (0.5 mL on either side).

Technique: A **peritendinous injection** is performed; both the anesthetic and corticosteroid are injected in a 1-inch-long linear track adjacent to the peritendinous thickening. Note: Never inject into the body of the tendon! The optimal injection is accomplished by inserting the needle from the most inferior point to the most superior point of the thickening and then slowly withdrawing the needle inferiorly, leaving a track of medication parallel to the tendon. If local tenderness is significantly relieved and dorsiflexion strength is unquestionably normal, then 0.5 mL of D80 is injected similarly. The entire sequence is repeated on the opposite side of the tendon. Even though

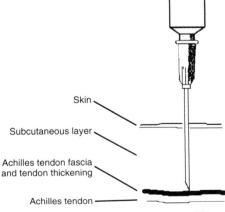

Skin

Subcutaneous layer

Achilles tendon fascia
and tendon thickening

Achilles tendon

Figure 10-3B Achilles tendinitis injection.

159

the peritendinous thickening often affects the medial aspect of the tendon more often, injection is still performed in equal amounts on either side of the tendon.

INJECTION AFTERCARE

1. Immobilization in a short-leg walking cast or air cast for 3 to 4 weeks is strongly recommended after local injection; casting protects the tendon from rupture following injection.
2. Crutches with touch-down weightbearing for the first few days are also strongly recommended, especially if an air cast is chosen.
3. *Acetaminophen* (1000 mg twice a day) is used for postinjection soreness.
4. During the recovery phase, jumping, twisting, and impact must be avoided.
5. *Passive stretching* of the ankle in flexion and extension is begun after the cast is removed—first by hand and then with progressive wall stretches.
6. The walking stride must be kept short while in the recovery phase.
7. The tendon must be protected from friction with the use of high-top shoes with padding over the tendon (double socks, felt ring, or mole foam).
8. *Isometric toning exercises* of ankle eversion and inversion are begun after flexibility has been partially restored and followed by isometric toning of the ankle in plantar flexion.
9. Request an *MRI* and a *consultation* with a surgical orthopedist if injection combined with immobilization fail to resolve the active tendinitis.

OUTCOME AND FURTHER WORK-UP: Achilles tendinitis treated in the first several months responds to rest, immobilization, and stretching exercises. Patients with long-standing symptoms (more than 4 to 6 months), tendon thickening more than two or three times normal in width, and those with a history of trauma require strict immobilization for longer periods, require more intense physical therapy recovery exercises, and have a greater risk of partial tendon tear. Patients with these risk factors should undergo MRI to determine the integrity of the tendon.

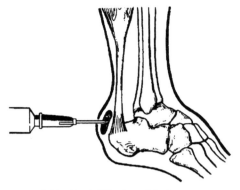

Enter over the posterior-superior aspect of the calcaneus, directly in the midline
Needle: $^5/_8$-inch, 25-gauge
Depth: $^1/_4$ to $^3/_8$ inch
Volume: 0.5 to 1 mL of anesthetic and 0.5 mL D80
NOTE: The injection should be superficial to the tendon; high pressure when injecting suggests an intratendinous position

Figure 10-4A Pre-Achilles bursa injection.

SUMMARY

Pre-Achilles bursitis is an inflammation of the bursal sac located between the calcaneal insertion of the Achilles tendon and the overlying skin. Its function is to reduce the friction between the skin and the tendon caused by poorly fitted or tight shoes. Although frequently misdiagnosed as Achilles tendinitis, it is distinctly different in pathology, location, and response to treatment. The local tenderness and inflammation of pre-Achilles bursitis is located directly over the calcaneus. By contrast, the tenderness and tendon thickening of Achilles tendinitis is located $1^1/_2$ inches above the calcaneus. Chronic irritation of the bursa can lead to calcification just posterior to the calcaneus. Achilles tendon rupture rarely occurs at this site.

TREATMENT OF CHOICE: Measures to reduce friction over the back of the heel (a large felt ring, moleskin, New-Skin, "V-notched" tennis shoes, or padded heel cups) combined with open-back shoes are the treatments of choice.

SEQUENCE OF TREATMENTS

1. Mildly symptomatic bursitis responds to ice, shortening of the stride, reducing friction over the tendon (double socks, mole foam, New-Skin, heel cups, or adhesive pads), and gradual tendon stretching.
2. *Injection:* Moderate to severe cases can be treated with corticosteroid injection (D80) combined with an air cast or a short-leg walking cast for 3 weeks (see details on page 162).
3. *Recovery exercise:* Passive Achilles tendon stretches are begun after the acute swelling and inflammation have resolved.
4. *Consultation:* Surgical consultation is indicated for large calcifications or refractory symptoms.
5. Full activities must be delayed until all signs of irritation have resolved and full flexibility restored.

SURGICAL PROCEDURE: The bony prominence of a large calcaneal calcification can be excised if associated with chronic irritation.

INJECTION: Local injection with anesthetic is often used to confirm the diagnosis and combined with corticosteroid to effectively arrest local inflammation. Injection combined with fixed immobilization (air or walking cast) improves the chances of a favorable outcome in severe or recurrent cases.

Position: The patient is placed in the prone position with the foot over the edge of the examination table. The ankle is kept in neutral position.

Surface Anatomy and the Point of Entry: The insertion of the Achilles tendon on the calcaneus is identified. The point of entry is in the midline, directly over the superior portion of the calcaneus, at the site of the distal attachment of the tendon.

Angle of Entry and Depth: The angle of entry is perpendicular to the skin. The depth is located at the interface of the dermis and the firm to hard resistance of the tendon insertion, approximately $\frac{1}{4}$ to $\frac{3}{8}$ inch from skin.

Anesthesia: Ethyl chloride is sprayed on the skin. Local anesthetic is placed just under the skin in the subcutaneous tissue (0.25 mL) and just posterior to the tendon (0.25 to 0.5 mL).

Technique: A **special pressure technique** is used to identify the bursal sac accurately. The skin is puckered in the midline to facilitate entry of the needle. The needle is advanced down to the firm to hard tissue resistance of the tendon (felt with the needle tip as increased tissue resistance or as increased pressure when attempting to inject anesthetic). With a constant, moderate injection pressure, the needle is very slowly withdrawn until the anesthetic flows easily. A proper placement should create a visible bulge the size of a dime. Note: The bursa will accept only small volumes! Use the least amount of anesthetic to confirm the diagnosis. Then reexamine the patient. If the local tenderness is significantly relieved, inject 0.5 mL of D80. Firm to hard pressure on injection suggests an intratendinous injection!

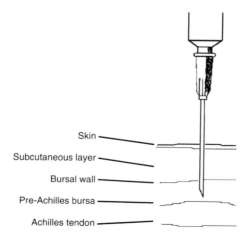

Skin

Subcutaneous layer

Bursal wall

Pre-Achilles bursa

Achilles tendon

Figure 10-4B   Pre-Achilles bursa injection.

INJECTION AFTERCARE

1. The ankle must be *protected for the first 3 days* by avoiding all unnecessary weightbearing (it takes 3 days for the medication to set up).
2. Lace-up high-top shoes with generous heel padding (double socks, felt ring, or mole foam) are recommended to protect the heel from direct pressure.
3. *Ice* (15 minutes every 4 to 6 hours), *acetaminophen* (1000 mg twice a day), or both, are used for postinjection soreness.
4. Movement of the ankle must be *restricted* for 3 to 4 weeks by avoiding all unnecessary walking and standing.
5. Shortening the stride reduces the pressure over the heel.
6. *Passive stretching* of the ankle in flexion and extension are begun after the pain and swelling have resolved.
7. *Injection* with corticosteroid can be repeated at 6 weeks if swelling recurs or pain persists.
8. *Plain film radiographs* are obtained and a *consultation* with a surgical orthopedist can be considered if two consecutive injections fail and the patient still complains of pain and swelling.

OUTCOME AND FURTHER WORK-UP: Local corticosteroid injection combined with padding over the back of the heel has a uniformly good prognosis. Patients that fail to experience long-term relief from local injection should have plain film radiographs of the ankle to evaluate the integrity of the calcaneus and to determine the presence of Achilles tendon calcification. Patients with calcaneal spurs exceeding 1 cm have a guarded prognosis and are more likely to require surgery.

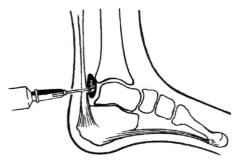

Enter from the lateral side of the
Achilles tendon, 1 inch above the
calcaneus
Needle: $1\frac{1}{2}$-inch, 22-gauge
Depth: $\frac{3}{4}$ to 1 inch ($\frac{1}{2}$ inch posterior
to the tibia and talus)
Volume: 0.5 mL of anesthetic and
0.5 mL K40
NOTE: Place the medication adjacent
to the talus rather than the Achilles
tendon

Figure 10-5A   Retrocalcaneal bursa injection.

SUMMARY

Retrocalcaneal bursitis—a minor bursa located between the Achilles tendon and the posterior aspect of the ankle—is an uncommon problem. Its function is to lubricate the tendon and the talus bone when the foot is in extreme plantar flexion. Symptoms consist of a vague posterior heel pain aggravated by extreme plantar flexion. The diagnosis is suggested by fullness in the space behind the ankle and local tenderness in the soft tissue space between the Achilles tendon and the ankle, and is confirmed by a regional anesthetic block placed in the bursa. The differential diagnosis includes calcaneal stress fracture, arthritis of the ankle, and tarsal tunnel syndrome.

TREATMENT OF CHOICE: Because NSAIDs are uniformly ineffective, local corticosteroid injection with K40 is the treatment of choice.

SEQUENCE OF TREATMENTS
1. *Injection:* Local anesthetic injection is used to accurately confirm the diagnosis, and corticosteroid (K40) is used to treat the active inflammation (see details on page 165).
2. A shortened walking stride limits the dorsiflexion of the ankle.
3. *Acute restrictions:* Impact, pivoting, stair climbing, and repetitive motion at the ankle must be limited.
4. *Most common immobilizer:* Padded heel cups help reduce the effects of impact.
5. *Recovery exercises:* Passive range of motion exercises of the ankle and Achilles tendon stretches are performed if the ankle flexibility has been diminished.

SURGICAL PROCEDURE: None.

INJECTION: Local injection with anesthetic is used to confirm the diagnosis and to differentiate this soft tissue condition from ankle arthritis, calcaneal bony lesions, tarsal tunnel, and so forth. Local corticosteroid is the preferred anti-inflammatory treatment.

Position: The patient is placed in the prone position with the foot hanging over the end of the examination table. The ankle is kept in neutral position.

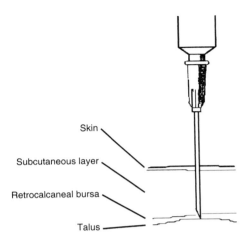

Skin

Subcutaneous layer

Retrocalcaneal bursa

Talus

Figure 10-5B Retrocalcaneal bursa injection.

Surface Anatomy and the Point of Entry: The Achilles tendon, the superior portion of the calcaneus, and the posterior aspect of the ankle are identified and marked. The point of entry is lateral to the Achilles tendon, 1 inch above the calcaneus.

Angle of Entry and Depth: The needle is angled from the lateral aspect of the Achilles tendon toward the center and midline of the talus. The depth is approximately 1 inch.

Anesthesia: Ethyl chloride is sprayed on the skin. Local anesthetic is placed in the subcutaneous tissue (0.5 mL) and just posterior to the talus (0.5 mL).

Technique: A **lateral approach** is used to avoid the neurovascular bundle of the foot; the posterior tibialis artery and nerve are located medially. The needle is advanced down to the hard resistance of the talus. Local anesthetic is injected just posterior to the talus and the patient reexamined. If local tenderness and pain with forced plantar flexion are relieved, 0.5 mL of K40 is injected.

INJECTION AFTERCARE

1. The ankle must be *protected for the first 3 days* by avoiding all unnecessary weight bearing.
2. Lace-up high-top shoes with generous heel padding (double socks, felt ring, or mole foam) are recommended to protect the heel from direct pressure.
3. *Ice* (15 minutes every 4 to 6 hours), *acetaminophen* (1000 mg twice a day), or both, are used for postinjection soreness.
4. Movement of the ankle must be *restricted* for 3 to 4 weeks by avoiding all unnecessary walking and standing.
5. Shortening the stride reduces the pressure over the heel.
6. *Passive stretching exercises* of the ankle in flexion and extension are begun after the pain and swelling have resolved.
7. *Injection* with corticosteroid can be repeated at 6 weeks if swelling recurs or pain persists.

165

8. *Plain film radiographs* are obtained to evaluate for subtle ankle arthritis and a *consultation* with a surgical orthopedist can be considered if two consecutive injections fail and the patient still complains of pain and swelling.

OUTCOME AND FURTHER WORK-UP: Local corticosteroid injection is highly efficacious for retrocalcaneal bursitis. Stretching and strengthening exercises of the Achilles tendon decrease the likelihood of a recurrence. If symptoms and signs persist, subtle abnormalities of the ankle joint (pronation, arthritis, or tarsal coalition), talus (subtalar arthritis or talar dome osteochondritis dissecans), or calcaneus (bony lesions) need to be excluded.

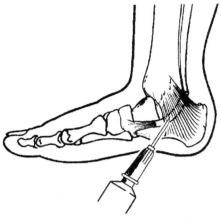

Enter just below the posterior edge of
  medial malleolus
Needle: $5/_8$-inch, 25-gauge
Depth: $3/_8$ to $1/_2$ inch
Volume: 1 to 2 mL anesthetic and
  0.5 mL D80
NOTE: Keep the bevel of the needle
  parallel to the tendon

Figure 10-6A   Posterior tibialis tendon injection.

SUMMARY
Posterior tibialis tenosynovitis is an inflammation of the medial ankle's tendon that inverts the foot and curves around the medial malleolus. It lies in a tenosynovial sheath that provides lubrication, reducing tendon friction as it rounds the medial malleolus. The patient complains of medial ankle pain. The examination consists of local tenderness and swelling just under the medial malleolus, pain aggravated by resisted inversion and plantar flexion, and pain aggravated by passively stretching the ankle in eversion. Ankle pronation, pes planus, ankle arthritis, and obesity are predisposing factors.

TREATMENT OF CHOICE: Initial treatment focuses on improving the alignment of the ankle (pes planus or ankle pronation) and any degree of ankle arthritis.

SEQUENCE OF TREATMENTS
1. *Injection:* Local anesthetic injection is used to confirm the diagnosis and distinguish tenosynovitis from involvement of the ankle or its supporting ligaments.
2. Shortening the walking stride reduces the tension across the tendon.
3. *Acute restriction:* Impact and repetitive motion at the ankle must be avoided.
4. *Most common immobilizer:* Depending on the severity, immobilization of the ankle with high-top shoes, a Velcro ankle brace, an air cast, or a short-leg walking cast can be used.
5. *Injection:* Local corticosteroid injection with D80 is indicated for persistent symptoms (see details on page 168).
6. *Recovery exercises:* Passive range of motion exercises of the ankle combined with isometric toning of inversion and eversion complete the recovery.

SURGICAL PROCEDURE: None.

INJECTION: Local injection with anesthetic can be used to confirm the diagnosis and to differentiate this soft tissue condition from subtalar arthritis. Local corticosteroid is indicated for persistent symptoms that fail to respond to correction of ankle alignment, arch abnormalities, and ankle immobilization.

Position: The patient is placed in the supine position. The leg is kept straight and the lower leg is externally rotated.

Surface Anatomy and the Point of Entry: The tip of the medial malleolus is identified. The needle is inserted just behind the posterior edge of the bone.

Angle of Entry and Depth: The needle is inserted perpendicular to the skin and is advanced to the firm resistance of the tendon ($\frac{3}{8}$ inch) or the hard resistance of the bone ($\frac{1}{2}$ inch).

Anesthesia: Ethyl chloride is sprayed on the skin. Local anesthetic is placed in the subcutaneous tissue (0.5 mL) and at the firm resistance of the tendon (0.5 mL).

Technique: An **intratenosynovial** injection is the aim of this technique. It can be performed in two ways. If the firm resistance of the tendon is easily identified as the needle is advanced, the injection can be placed at this site. However, if the tendon is not readily identified, the needle is advanced down to the hard resistance of the bone and then withdrawn $\frac{1}{8}$ inch. Note: As the needle is advanced to the bone, the bevel must be kept parallel to the course of the tendon fibers. The pressure of injection will be minimal if the needle is in the tenosynovial sheath. Finally, if local tenderness and isometric pain with resisted ankle inversion are improved, then 0.5 mL D80 is injected.

INJECTION AFTERCARE
1. The ankle must be *protected for the first 3 days* by avoiding all unnecessary weightbearing.
2. Lace-up high-top shoes, an air cast, or a short-leg walking cast is recommended depending on the severity of the tendinitis and the associated pronation, arthritis, and so forth.
3. *Ice* (15 minutes every 4 to 6 hours), *acetaminophen* (1000 mg twice a day), or both, are used for postinjection soreness.

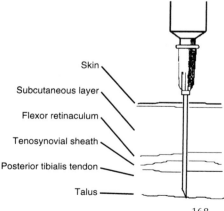

Skin
Subcutaneous layer
Flexor retinaculum
Tenosynovial sheath
Posterior tibialis tendon
Talus

Figure 10-6B Posterior tibialis tendon injection.

168

4. Movement of the ankle must be *restricted* for 3 to 4 weeks by limiting all unnecessary walking and standing.
5. Shortening the stride reduces the stress on the tendon.
6. *Passive stretching* of the ankle in flexion and extension are begun after the pain and swelling have resolved.
7. *Injection* with corticosteroid can be repeated at 6 weeks if swelling recurs or pain persists.
8. *Isometric toning exercises* of ankle inversion and eversion are begun once flexibility has been partially restored.
9. *Plain film radiographs* are obtained to evaluate for subtle ankle arthritis, and a *consultation* with a surgical orthopedist can be considered if two consecutive injections fail and the patient still complains of pain and swelling.

OUTCOME AND FURTHER WORK-UP: Posterior tibialis tendinitis most often results from biomechanical stresses of ankle pronation, abnormalities of the arch, or ankle arthritis. Long-term success depends on the correction of these associated conditions. Surgery is usually reserved for tendon rupture, a rare event.

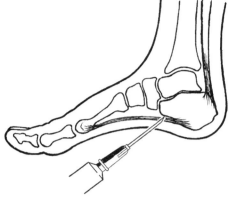

Enter through the plantar surface in
the midline ³/₄-inch distal to the
origin of the plantar fascia
Needle: 1¹/₂-inch, 22-gauge
Depth: 1 to 1¹/₂ inches
Volume: 1 to 2 mL anesthetic and
1 mL D80
NOTE: The injection must be at a
depth greater than 1 inch to avoid
injecting steroid in the specialized
fat of the heel pad!

Figure 10-7A   Plantar fascial injection.

SUMMARY

Plantar fasciitis is an inflammation of the origin of the longitudinal ligament, the principal
ligament that forms the arch of the foot. Flat feet (pes planus), high arches (pes cavus), turned-in
ankles (ankle pronation), and tight Achilles tendons predispose to the condition. Obesity, working
on concrete, poorly fitted shoes, and prolonged daily standing aggravate the condition. A few cases
are purely inflammatory in nature and are associated with Reiter's syndrome. The patient
complains of local tenderness at or just medial to the origin of the plantar fascia. By contrast,
patients diagnosed with heel pad syndrome complain of diffuse heel pain and demonstrate diffuse
heel tenderness, and patients with calcaneal fracture, calcaneal stress fracture, or Sever's
epiphysitis complain of diffuse heel pain that can be reproduced by side-to-side compression of
the calcaneus on examination.

TREATMENT OF CHOICE: Initial treatment should always start with padded arch supports
and correction of ankle pronation.

SEQUENCE OF TREATMENTS
1. Padded arch supports must be worn continuously in well-fitted shoes.
2. *Acute restrictions:* Tiptoeing or pressure across the ball of the feet (stairs, pedals, exercise
    equipment, etc.) must be avoided completely and in severe cases combined with restricted
    weight bearing.
3. *Exercise of choice:* Progressive Achilles tendon stretching is performed by hand pressure
    initially, then followed by wall stretches as flexibility is regained.
4. Ice massaged over the bottom of the heel relieves pain and reduces the irritation of the first few
    steps in the morning.
5. *Most common immobilizer:* Taping of the ankle and the arch is a time-honored method of
    supporting the arch.

6. *Injection:* Local corticosteroid injection with D80 is combined with immobilization using high-top shoes with soft arch supports in place.

7. *Injection* can be repeated at 4 to 6 weeks but should be combined with immobilization using either an air cast or short-leg walking cast for greater protection.

8. Custom-made arch supports may be required for the patient with dramatic degrees of pes planus or pes cavus.

9. *Consultation:* Surgical consultation can be considered if two injections combined with immobilization fail to resolve the condition.

SURGICAL PROCEDURE: Fascial débridement with or without calcaneal spur removal is the most common procedure performed.

INJECTION: Treatment focuses on padding the heel (heel cups, heel cushions, or padded insoles), supporting the arch (padded arch supports, and well-supporting shoes), and performing daily Achilles tendon stretching exercises. Local injection with corticosteroids is indicated for persistent symptoms. Difficult cases may require two injections and rigid immobilization.

Position: The patient is placed in the prone position with the foot hanging just off the edge of the examination table.

Surface Anatomy and the Point of Entry: The inferior surface of the calcaneus and the origin of the plantar fascia (approximately 1 to $1\frac{1}{2}$ inches from the back of the heel) are identified. The point of entry is $\frac{3}{4}$ inch **distal** to the origin of the fascia in the midline.

Angle of Entry and Depth: The needle is inserted at a 45-degree angle and is advanced to the firm resistance of the fascia (1 inch) and then onto the hard resistance of the bone ($1\frac{1}{2}$ inches).

Anesthesia: Ethyl chloride is sprayed on the skin. Local anesthetic is placed in the subcutaneous tissue (0.5 mL), intradermally (0.25 mL), at the firm resistance of the fascia (0.5 mL), and in between the fascia and the calcaneus (0.5 mL).

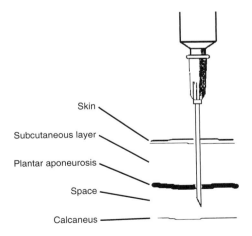

Skin

Subcutaneous layer

Plantar aponeurosis

Space

Calcaneus

Figure 10-7B Plantar fascial injection.

171

Technique: In order to accurately inject between the plantar fascia and the calcaneus and hence avoid injecting into the specialized fat of the heel pad, a **plantar approach** is strongly suggested. Generous anesthetic is given at the plantar surface. The needle is then advanced through the low-resistance fat to the subtle to firm resistance of the fascia. A popping or "giving way" is often felt when passing through the fascia. Caution: The patient may experience pain as the periosteum of the calcaneus is touched. If the local tenderness is significantly relieved, 1 mL of D80 is injected slowly. Caution: The space is small; the rapid injection of medication can be painful!

INJECTION AFTERCARE

1. The fascia must be *protected for the first 3 days* by avoiding all unnecessary weightbearing.
2. Lace-up high-top shoes, an air cast, or a short-leg walking cast is recommended depending on the severity of the fasciitis and the associated pronation, arthritis, and so forth.
3. *Ice* (15 minutes every 4 to 6 hours), *acetaminophen* (1000 mg twice a day), or both, are used for postinjection soreness.
4. The forces placed across the fascia must be *restricted* for 3 to 4 weeks by limiting all unnecessary walking and standing.
5. Shortening the stride reduces the stress on the fascia.
6. *Passive stretching exercises* of the ankle in flexion and extension are begun after the pain and swelling have resolved.
7. *Injection* with corticosteroid can be repeated at 6 weeks if pain recurs or persists and is combined with immobilization to enhance the response.
8. Request a *consultation* with a surgical orthopedist or podiatrist if two consecutive injections and fixed immobilization fail.

OUTCOME AND FURTHER WORK-UP: Plantar fasciitis results from the biomechanic stresses caused by tight Achilles tendons, ankle pronation, and abnormalities of the arch. Treatment that is directed at the plantar fascia, Achilles tendon, arch, and ankle will guarantee the optimal outcome. Patients with large "heel spurs"—$\frac{1}{2}$ inch or longer—are at greater risk of treatment failure or recurrent symptoms. Early surgical consultation can be considered in these cases.

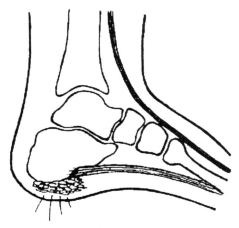

Treatment of choice is padded heel
cups
Calcaneus
Specialized fat of the heel
Plantar fascia

Figure 10-8   Heel pad syndrome.

SUMMARY

Traumatic irritation of the specialized fat that covers and protects the calcaneus is referred to as "heel pad syndrome." The diagnosis is suggested by a history of trauma, diffuse tenderness over the entire heel, pain aggravated by squeezing the fat pad from either side, and an absence of focal bony tenderness (calcaneal fracture or plantar fasciitis). Radiographic studies are normal. The goal of treatment is to reduce the direct pressure over the fat pad, allowing the tissues to heal and to return to normal.

TREATMENT OF CHOICE: Heel cups or padded insoles are used to reduce the direct pressure over the heel.

SEQUENCE OF TREATMENTS

1.   *Most common immobilizer:* Heel cups or padded arch supports worn continuously for 1 to 2 weeks in well-fitted shoes provide the most effective protection.
2.   *Restrictions:* Weightbearing must be limited, ranging from reduced walking, standing, and avoiding hard surfaces to using crutches for the first few days.
3.   A fatigue mat to stand on is an additional means to guard against direct pressure.
4.   Ice over the heel in the first few days is an effective analgesic.
5.   *Recovery exercises:* Passive range of motion exercises of the ankle and Achilles tendon are appropriate recovery exercises if treatment has led to a reduced flexibility of the ankle.

SURGICAL PROCEDURE: None.

OUTCOME AND FURTHER WORK-UP: Patients with an uncomplicated heel pad syndrome should resolve their symptoms and signs within 2 to 3 weeks when treated with proper padding of the heel. Patients with persistent symptoms should be evaluated for subtle injury to the calcaneus (stress fracture or nondisplaced fractures), plantar fasciitis, or subtalar joint inflammation.

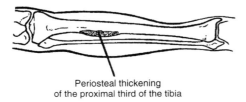

Periosteal thickening
of the proximal third of the tibia

Figure 10-9   Tibial stress fracture.

SUMMARY
Stress fractures of the tibia result from repeated microtrauma to the proximal third of the bone, often occurring in the section of the tibia with the smallest cross-sectional area. The condition is seen almost exclusively in runners, professional ballet dancers, and military recruits, although patients with severe osteoporotic bones are also susceptible. Radiographically, the periosteum of the tibia is thickened in the proximal third of the bone in runners as compared with the middle third of the bone in ballet dancers. A true fracture line is seen rarely. Stress fracture must be distinguished from the more common shin splints, anterior compartment syndrome, and localized pain or paresthesia of the outer lower leg caused by lumbosacral radiculopathy.

TREATMENT OF CHOICE: Running and walking must be curtailed until the pain and the radiographic changes are improved or at least stabilized.

SEQUENCE OF TREATMENTS
1. *Acute restrictions:* Running and other impact types of sports must be reduced for several weeks, with crutches recommended for those patients with severe pain.
2. *Most common immobilizer:* Persistent cases may require fixed immobilization with an air cast or short-leg walking cast.
3. *Exercise of choice:* Nonimpact muscle toning exercises can be continued.
4. Padded arch supports are worn continuously in well-fitted shoes for prevention.

SURGICAL PROCEDURE: None.

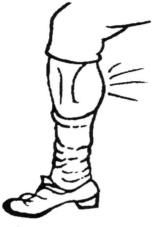

Any of the muscles of the posterior leg can be severely strained or partially torn; the posterior leg muscles include
At the Knee:
Semimembranosus
Semitendinosus
Biceps femoris
Plantaris
Popliteus
In the Calf:
Soleus
Gastrocnemius

Figure 10-10   Gastrocnemius muscle tear.

SUMMARY

Gastrocnemius muscle tears usually occur in the proximal third of the muscle and are nearly always a result of trauma. Pain and tenderness are typically focal. A palpable defect in the muscle accompanies the larger tears. Bleeding or bruising is typically not apparent initially and rarely at the site of injury. Bleeding dissects down the leg along the tissue planes to the ankle, forming the classic crescent sign at the malleolus. This soft tissue injury must be distinguished from a ruptured Baker's cyst and lower extremity deep venous thrombosis.

TREATMENT OF CHOICE: Weightbearing is either restricted or avoided depending on the severity of the injury. This is followed by reduced walking, running, stair climbing, and jumping.

SEQUENCE OF TREATMENTS
1. Deep venous thrombosis must be excluded in patients with significant risk factors for thrombosis.
2. *Acute restrictions:* Running, walking, prolonged standing, and other weightbearing activities must be restricted for 1 to 3 weeks.
3. Crutches may be necessary in the first week.
4. *Most common immobilizer:* An Ace wrap or athletic taping is combined with ice applications in the first few days.
5. *Recovery exercises:* Passive stretching of the ankle in dorsiflexion is followed by a gradual return to regular activities.

INJECTION: None.

SURGICAL PROCEDURE: None.

Chapter 11

FOOT

THE DIFFERENTIAL DIAGNOSIS OF FOOT PAIN

DIAGNOSES	CONFIRMATIONS
Anatomy	
Pes planus and pes cavus	Examination
Metatarsalgia	
Tight extensor tendons or hammer toe deformity (most common)	Examination
Morton's neuroma	Local anesthetic block
Rheumatoid arthritis	Examination; rheumatoid factor
Corns and calluses	Examination
Plantar warts	Examination
First metatarsophalangeal (MTP) joint	
Osteoarthritis	
Bunion	Radiographs: foot series
Hallux rigidus	Radiographs: foot series
Prebunion bursa	Local anesthetic block
Gout (podagra)	Synovial fluid analysis
Sesamoiditis	Radiographs: sesamoid view
Swelling over the dorsum of the foot	
Extensor tenosynovitis	Examination
Cellulitis	Examination; complete blood count
Stress fracture of the metatarsals	Radiographs; bone scanning
Reflex sympathetic dystrophy	Bone scanning
Dorsal bunion	Radiographs: foot series
Bunionette of the fifth MTP joint	Examination; radiographs: foot series
Referred pain	
Lumbosacral spine radiculopathy	Computed tomography (CT) scan; magnetic resonance imaging (MRI); electromyogram (EMG)
Tarsal tunnel syndrome	Nerve conduction velocity testing

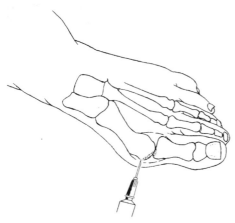

Enter over the MTP joint medially at
the distal metatarsal head
Needle: $\frac{5}{8}$-inch, 25-gauge
Depth: $\frac{1}{4}$ to $\frac{3}{8}$ inch (flush against the
bone)
Volume: 0.5 mL anesthetic and
0.25 mL K40
NOTE: The injection is made under the
synovial membrane adjacent to the
bone, not in between the articular
surfaces of the joint

Figure 11-1A   First metatarsophalangeal (MTP) joint (bunion) injection.

SUMMARY

"Bunion" is the term used to describe to the bony prominence and abnormal angle of the great toe, the hallmark of osteoarthritis of the first MTP joint. Asymmetric pressure over the articular cartilage caused by narrow-toebox shoes leads to the accelerated wear of the articular cartilage, subsequent angulation of the joint, and gradual subluxation of the extensor tendons. The wear-and-tear effect on the joint leads to the typical valgus deformity. Continued pressure over the medial joint line can cause acute arthritic flares or acute adventitial bursitis. The goals of treatment are to protect the joint from pressure and impact, realign the deformity, and prevent any further arthritic change and deformity.

TREATMENT OF CHOICE: Emphasis is always placed on wearing wide-toebox shoes with adhesive padding over the medial MTP joint.

SEQUENCE OF TREATMENTS
1. Wide-toebox shoes are mandatory.
2. Adhesive bunion pad (felt ring) or bunion shield is worn inside the shoe.
3. Padded insoles worn continuously protect the joint against pressure from below.
4. *Acute restrictions:* Weightbearing activities must be limited, such as walking and standing.
5. Shortening the stride decreases the motion across the joint.
6. *Injection:* Corticosteroid injection with triamcinolone acetonide 40 mg/mL (K40) is used for the acute arthritic flares (see details on page 179).
7. *Exercise of choice:* Passive stretching of the MTP joint is used to maintain flexibility and is performed after the acute symptoms have resolved.
8. *Consultation:* Surgical consultation is reserved for advanced disease or at the patient's insistence.

SURGICAL PROCEDURE: Bunionectomy—bony osteotomy, joint realignment, and extensor tendon release—attempts to restore the normal appearance of the great toe.

INJECTION: Treatment focuses on protecting the joint from pressure against the medial and inferior surfaces. Local corticosteroid injection is used to control the symptoms of an acute inflammatory flare and to provide temporary relief for this progressive arthritic condition.

Position: The patient is placed in the supine position with the leg extended and the foot externally rotated.

Surface Anatomy and the Point of Entry: The head of the first metatarsal (the medial prominence) and the medial MTP joint line are palpated and marked. The point of entry is adjacent to the joint line, approximately $\frac{1}{4}$ inch distal to the prominence.

Angle of Entry and Depth: The needle is inserted perpendicular to the skin and is advanced to the hard resistance of the bone ($\frac{1}{4}$ to $\frac{3}{8}$ inch).

Anesthesia: Ethyl chloride is sprayed on the skin. Local anesthetic is placed in the subcutaneous tissue (0.25 mL) and just outside the synovial membrane at $\frac{1}{4}$ inch (0.25 mL). All anesthetic should be injected outside the joint. The intra-articular injection is reserved for corticosteroids because the joint accepts only small volumes!

Technique: A **medial approach** to the joint's synovial membrane is safest and easiest to perform. After placing the anesthetic just outside the synovial membrane, the first syringe is replaced with a second syringe containing the corticosteroid. Then the needle is advanced down to the periosteum of the bone. If the tip of the needle rests against the metatarsal bone, the injection will flow under the synovial membrane and into the joint. Gentle pressure is required. Note: The needle is *not* advanced into the center of the joint!

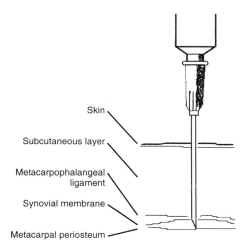

Skin

Subcutaneous layer

Metacarpophalangeal ligament

Synovial membrane

Metacarpal periosteum

Figure 11-1B   Bunion injection.

INJECTION AFTERCARE

1. The toe must be *protected for the first 3 days* by avoiding all unnecessary weightbearing.
2. Loose fitting, wide-toebox shoes with extra padding (double socks, felt ring, or mole foam) are combined with a padded insole.
3. A toe spacer (cotton, foam) is used to improve alignment.
4. *Ice* (15 minutes every 4 to 6 hours), *acetaminophen (Tylenol ES)* (1000 mg twice a day), or both, are used for postinjection soreness.
5. Movement of the toe must be *restricted* for 3 to 4 weeks by avoiding all unnecessary walking and standing.
6. Shortening the stride reduces the stress on the toe.
7. *Passive stretching* exercises of the toe in flexion and extension are begun after the pain and swelling have been controlled.
8. *Injection* can be repeated at 6 weeks with corticosteroid if pain recurs or persists.
9. *Plain film radiographs* of the foot are obtained and a *consultation* with a surgical orthopedist or podiatrist is considered if two consecutive injections fail to control pain and swelling.

OUTCOME AND FURTHER WORK-UP: The long-term outcome is solely dependent on wearing the appropriate shoes with sufficient padding to protect against the pressure and impact of walking. Plain film radiographs are very useful in defining the severity of the osteoarthritic changes affecting the great toe and the appropriateness of surgical referral.

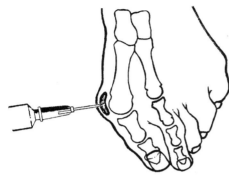

Enter the bursal sac medially over the
    point of maximum swelling (over
    the distal head of the metatarsal)
Needle: $^5/_8$-inch, 25-gauge
Depth: $^1/_4$ to $^3/_8$ inch ($^1/_8$ inch above
    the bone)
Volume: 0.5 to 1 mL anesthetic and
    0.25 K40
NOTE: The bursa lies between
    the subcutaneous fat layer and the
    synovial membrane

Figure 11-2A   Injection of the adventitial bursa over the first metatarsophalangeal joint.

SUMMARY

The constant pressure and friction of tight shoes over the medial aspect of the first MTP joint causes a bursal sac to develop. Further repetitive pressure and friction cause the bursal sac to become acutely inflamed. The swelling, redness, and tenderness are so dramatic that the condition is often misdiagnosed as acute gout. However, the inflammation is restricted to the medial aspect of the joint, in contrast to the inflammation of acute gout that encompasses the entire joint. The goals of treatment are to reduce the acute inflammation and to protect the metatarsal from pressure.

TREATMENT OF CHOICE: The key to treatment is protecting the medial side of the joint from direct pressure and friction by wearing wide-toebox shoes and an adhesive padding placed over the bursa.

SEQUENCE OF TREATMENTS

1. Wide-toebox shoes are mandatory.
2. ***Most common immobilizer:*** Adhesive bunion pads or a bunion shield is used to reduce direct pressure and friction.
3. Ice over the medial joint is very effective in controlling pain and swelling.
4. ***Injection:*** Local corticosteroid injection with K40 should be considered early if swelling and inflammation are dramatic (see details on page 182).
5. Shortening the stride is effective in reducing pressure and friction.
6. ***Consultation:*** Surgical consultation is considered for persistent symptoms.

SURGICAL PROCEDURE: Bursectomy is the treatment of choice but is usually performed during the course of bunionectomy.

INJECTION: Local anesthetic block is used to differentiate this periarticular condition from gout. Corticosteroid injection is used to control the symptoms of the acute inflammatory flare.

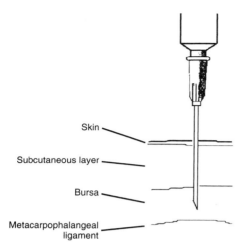

Skin

Subcutaneous layer

Bursa

Metacarpophalangeal
ligature

Figure 11-2B   Metatarsophalangeal
bursitis injection.

Position: The patient is placed in the supine position with the leg extended and the foot externally
rotated.

Surface Anatomy and the Point of Entry: The bursa lies directly over the medial prominence of
the MTP joint. The point of entry is directly over the center of the bursa.

Angle of Entry and Depth: The needle is inserted perpendicular to the skin. The depth is no
greater than $\frac{1}{4}$ to $\frac{3}{8}$ inch.

Anesthesia: Ethyl chloride is sprayed on the skin. Local anesthetic is placed in the subcutaneous
tissue (0.25 mL).

Technique: A **medial approach** is preferred. After anesthetic is placed, the needle is advanced
down to the hard resistance of the bone and then withdrawn $\frac{1}{4}$ inch (the bursa is located just
outside the capsule of the joint!). Attempts to aspirate fluid are usually unsuccessful. With the
needle held carefully in place 0.25 mL of K40 is injected.

INJECTION AFTERCARE

1. The toe must be ***protected for the first 3 days*** by avoiding all unnecessary weightbearing.
2. Loose fitting, wide-toebox shoes with extra padding (double socks, felt ring, or mole foam) are
    combined with a padded insole.
3. A toe spacer (cotton, foam) is used to improve alignment.
4. ***Ice*** (15 minutes every 4 to 6 hours), ***acetaminophen*** (1000 mg twice a day), or both, are used
    for postinjection soreness.
5. Movement of the toe must be ***restricted*** for 3 to 4 weeks by limiting unnecessary walking and
    standing.
6. Shortening the stride reduces the stress on the toe.
7. ***Passive stretching*** exercises of the toe in flexion and extension are begun after the pain and
    swelling have resolved.

8. *Injection* can be repeated at 6 weeks with corticosteroid if pain recurs or persists.
9. *Plain film radiographs* of the foot are obtained and a *consultation* with a surgical orthopedist or podiatrist can be considered if two consecutive injections fail to control pain and swelling.

OUTCOME AND FURTHER WORK-UP: Local corticosteroid injection is very effective in controlling the symptoms of the acute, inflammatory flare. Surgery is usually directed to the underlying bunion. Bursectomy without surgical correction of the underlying bunion deformity is usually ineffective.

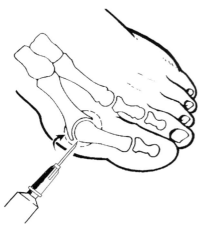

Enter medially either on the metatarsal or the phalangeal side of the joint line
Needle: $5/8$-inch, 25-gauge for anesthesia or 21-gauge for aspiration
Depth: $3/8$ to $1/2$ inch (depending on swelling)
Volume: 0.5 to 1 mL of anesthetic and 0.25 mL K40
NOTE: Multiple attempts to enter the joint may be damaging; with the needle flush against the periosteum—under the synovial membrane—the needle is intra-articular; manual pressure may yield sufficient fluid for analysis

Figure 11-3 Injection and aspiration of acute gout (podagra).

SUMMARY

Gout is an acute crystal induced, monarthric arthritis of the MTP joint of the great toe. Acute swelling, redness, and heat develop as an inflammatory response to the precipitation of monosodium urate crystals in the synovial fluid. The synovial fluid becomes supersaturated with uric acid crystals as a result of overproduction of uric acid (hemolytic anemia, leukemia, psoriasis, tumors with rapid cell turnover, and other causes of overproduction account for 10% of cases) or undersecretion of uric acid (diuretics, renal disease, aspirin, and niacin are the most common drugs that account for nearly 90% of cases). Patients with recurrent gouty attacks should undergo laboratory evaluation to determine the cause of their altered metabolism. Gout can also affect the olecranon and prepatellar bursa, the tenosynovial sheaths of the dorsum of the foot and instep, and the other small joints of the foot.

INJECTION: Corticosteroid injection is indicated when the nonsteroidal anti-inflammatory drugs (NSAIDs) are contraindicated (peptic ulcer disease, concurrent use of warfarin [Coumadin], renal failure, etc.). The general treatment of gout is very similar to the treatment of bunions (see page 179). Injection with local anesthetic is also used for aspirating the joint for crystal analysis (see later).

Special Technique: A **medial approach** to aspirate the joint is safest and easiest to perform. After placing the anesthetic just outside the synovial membrane, the needle is advanced to the periosteum of the metatarsal and 0.25 mL of anesthetic is placed under the synovial membrane. With the needle held carefully in place, gentle manual pressure is exerted over the lateral and medial aspects of the joint to express one or two drops of synovial fluid for crystal analysis. Leaving the needle in place, 0.5 mL of K40 is injected into the joint. Caution: Passing the needle into the center of the joint can be damaging.

184

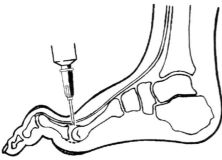

Enter from above, midway between
the MTP joints. After placing
anesthetic in the dermis, advance
the needle at a 45-degree angle
down to the periosteum of the
metatarsal head
Needle: ⅝-inch, 25-gauge
Depth: ⅜ to ½ inch to the periosteum
of the metatarsal head
Volume: 0.5 mL anesthetic and
0.25 mL K40

Figure 11-4A   Injection of the acutely inflamed metatarsophalangeal (MTP) joint as a part of hammer toes.

SUMMARY

Metatarsalgia is the term used to describe painful MTP joints. Hammer toes—the most common cause of metatarsalgia, which also includes bunions, gout, rheumatoid arthritis, and Morton's neuroma—is the end result of inflexible, contracted extensor tendons of the foot. As the tendons gradually lose their flexibility, the MTP joints gradually extend and the proximal interphalangeal (PIP) joints gradually flex. Eventually a hammer-like deformity results. Pressure over these joints causes the skin to thicken over the bony prominences. Calluses form on the plantar surfaces and hard corns on the dorsal surfaces.

TREATMENT OF CHOICE: Passive stretching of the dorsal extensor tendons of the toes is the treatment of choice for early metatarsalgia. However, once the classic hammer toe deformity develops, surgical correction is preferred.

SEQUENCE OF TREATMENTS

1. *Exercise of choice:* The dorsal extensor tendons of the toes are passively stretched in a downward direction (manual stretching, picking up marbles, or grasping a towel).
2. Wide-toebox shoes are mandatory.
3. *Most common immobilizer:* A hammer toe crest placed under the four MTP joints is used to correct the hammer toe deformity.
4. Padded insoles worn continuously are used to protect the MTP heads from developing calluses.
5. Other pressure-relieving treatments include adhesive corn pads, paring of thick plantar calluses, and a cotton ball taped in place between the two most affected toes.
6. *Acute restrictions:* Walking, standing, and other weightbearing activities must be restricted.
7. Shortening the stride decreases the motion and stress across the joints.
8. *Injection:* Corticosteroid injection with K40 for arthritic flares (see details on page 186).
9. *Consultation:* Surgical consultation is indicated for the severe, fixed deformity or at the patient's insistence.

SURGICAL PROCEDURE: Arthroplasty with or without fusion with K-wires is the most common procedure.

INJECTION: Treatment focuses on stretching exercises, padding, treatment of the secondary corns and calluses, and wide-toebox shoes. Local corticosteroid injection is most often indicated for the acute inflammatory flare localized to one or two joints.

Position: The patient is placed in the supine position with the leg extended and the foot plantar flexed.

Surface Anatomy and the Point of Entry: The heads of the MTP joints are palpated from above and below and marked. The point of entry is centered between the two MTP joint heads, approximately $\frac{1}{2}$ inch back from the web space.

Angle of Entry and Depth: The needle is inserted into the skin at a 45-degree angle and is directed toward the most affected joint. The depth to the synovial membrane is $\frac{3}{8}$ to $\frac{1}{2}$ inch.

Anesthesia: Ethyl chloride is sprayed on the skin. Local anesthetic is placed in the subcutaneous tissue (0.25 mL) and just outside the synovial membrane at $\frac{3}{8}$ inch (0.25 mL). All anesthetic should be kept outside the joint because it will hold only a small volume!

Technique: A **dorsal approach** to the MTP joint is preferred. The 25-gauge needle is introduced midway between the MTP joints and advanced at a 45-degree angle down to the bone of the metatarsal head (typically $\frac{1}{2}$ inch down). Anesthesia is placed just outside the synovial membrane. The first syringe is removed and is replaced with the syringe containing the corticosteroid. The needle is advanced to the periosteum, and with the needle held flush against the bone, 0.25 mL of K40 is injected. Note: An injection placed underneath the synovial membrane is an intra-articular injection.

INJECTION AFTERCARE
1. The toes must be ***protected for the first 3 days*** by avoiding all unnecessary weightbearing.
2. Loose fitting, wide-toebox shoes with extra padding (double socks, felt ring, or mole foam) are combined with a padded insole.

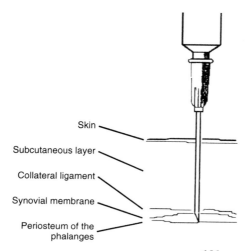

Skin

Subcutaneous layer

Collateral ligament

Synovial membrane

Periosteum of the phalanges

Figure 11-4B　Hammer toe injection.

3. A toe spacer (cotton, foam) is used to improve alignment and minimize pressure.
4. *Ice* (15 minutes every 4 to 6 hours), *acetaminophen* (1000 mg twice a day), or both, are used for postinjection soreness.
5. Movement of the toes must be *restricted* for 3 to 4 weeks by limiting all unnecessary walking and standing.
6. Shortening the stride reduces the stress on the toes.
7. *Passive stretching* exercises of the toes in flexion are begun at 3 to 4 weeks (manual stretching, picking up marbles, grasping a towel, or grabbing plush carpet).
8. *Injection* can be repeated at 6 weeks with corticosteroid if pain recurs or persists.
9. *Plain film radiographs* of the foot are obtained and a *consultation* with a surgical orthopedist or podiatrist can be considered if two consecutive injections fail to control pain and swelling, the PIP joints have fixed contractures, and the patient is willing to undergo possible fusion.

OUTCOME AND FURTHER WORK-UP: Daily stretching exercises of the dorsal extensor tendons when combined with wide-toebox shoes, padded insoles, hammer toe crests, and cotton or rubber toe spacers is the most effective treatment of hammer toes. The outcome is especially favorable when begun in the early stages of the condition, that is, before fixed contractures occur. Local injection is used infrequently. Plain film radiographs are used to evaluate for rheumatoid arthritis when symmetrical involvement of the MTP joints exists.

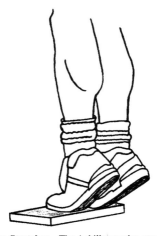

Figure 11-5 Achilles Tendon Stretches—The Achilles tendon stretching exercise is used to increase the flexibility of the ankle, reduce the traction exerted on the plantar fascia, reduce the recurrence of Achilles tendinitis, and protect the ankle joint against further injury. It is an advanced exercise compared with the classic Achilles tendon wall stretch. This exercise combines stretching of the tendon with strengthening of the gastrocnemius and soleus muscles. The wall stretch exercise should be mastered before advancing to this more demanding exercise.

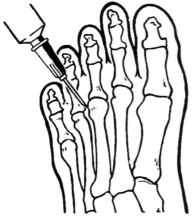

Enter from above, $^{1}/_{2}$ inch distal to the
  MTP joint
Needle: $^{5}/_{8}$-inch, 25-gauge
Depth: $^{5}/_{8}$ to $^{3}/_{4}$ inch (below the
  transverse metatarsal ligament)
Volume: 0.5 mL anesthetic and
  0.25 mL K40
NOTE: This injection is identical to a
  digital block

Figure 11-6A   Morton's neuroma injection. MTP, metatarsophalangeal.

SUMMARY

Morton's neuroma is a chronic irritation and inflammation of the digital nerve as it courses
between the MTP heads. Pressure from below (walking and standing on hard surfaces with poorly
padded shoes) and pressure from the sides (tight shoes) cause the nerve to enlarge gradually; the
pathologic changes consist of perineural thickening and fibrosis. The digital nerve located in the
web space between the third and fourth toes is affected most commonly.

TREATMENT OF CHOICE: Treatment should always emphasize reducing direct pressure with
either cotton or rubber toe spacers, padded insoles, or both, placed in wide-toebox shoes.

SEQUENCE OF TREATMENTS
1.   Wide-toebox shoes reduce the pressure from the sides.
2.   Padded insoles protect the nerve from pressure from below.
3.   *Most common immobilizer:* Commercially available toe spacers or cotton balls placed between
     two adjacent toes and held in place with tape keep the metatarsal heads apart.
4.   *Acute restrictions:* All unnecessary weightbearing must be restricted.
5.   The nerve can be protected by shortening the stride, decreasing the motion across the joints.
6.   *Injection:* Corticosteroid injection using K40 is used to reduce inflammation and perineural
     fibrosis (see details on page 189).
7.   *Consultation:* Surgical consultation can be considered if two injections 6 weeks apart fail to
     control symptoms

SURGICAL PROCEDURE: Neurectomy, surgical removal of the nerve, is the definitive surgical
procedure.

INJECTION: Local anesthetic injection is often used to confirm the diagnosis. Local corticosteroid injection is indicated when padding, protection, and change in shoes fail to control symptoms.

Position: The patient is placed in the supine position with the leg extended and the foot plantar flexed to 30 degrees.

Surface Anatomy and the Point of Entry: The heads of the MTP joints are palpated from above and below and marked. The point of entry is centered between the two MTP joint heads, approximately $\frac{1}{2}$ inch back from the web space.

Angle of Entry and Depth: The needle is inserted perpendicular to the skin and advanced down through the transverse tarsal ligament (between the metatarsal heads). The depth of is $\frac{3}{8}$ to $\frac{1}{2}$ inch to the transverse tarsal ligament and $\frac{5}{8}$ to $\frac{3}{4}$ inch to the nerve.

Anesthesia: Ethyl chloride is sprayed on the skin. Local anesthetic is placed in the subcutaneous tissue (0.25 mL), the transverse tarsal ligament (0.25 mL), and just below the ligament (0.25 to 0.5 mL). If the injection is placed accurately under the transverse tarsal ligament, the inner aspects of the adjacent toes should be numb!

Technique: A **dorsal approach** to the MTP joint is preferred. The proximal phalangeal heads are palpated. A 25-gauge needle is introduced halfway between the MTP heads and advanced to the firm resistance of the transverse tarsal ligament (subtle). Following anesthesia at this level, the needle is advanced through the ligament. Often a "giving way" or popping sensation is felt. At this point 0.25 to 0.5 mL of anesthetic is injected and the patient is reexamined. If local tenderness and MTP squeeze sign are relieved, 0.25 mL of K40 is injected.

INJECTION AFTERCARE

1. *Rest* for 3 days, avoiding all unnecessary weightbearing.
2. Recommend loose-fitting, wide-toebox shoes with extra padding (double socks, padded insoles, or padded arch supports when indicated).
3. Use a toe spacer to improve alignment and minimize pressure.

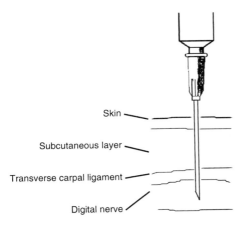

Skin

Subcutaneous layer

Transverse carpal ligament

Digital nerve

Figure 11-6B Morton's neuroma injection.

4.   *Ice* (15 minutes every 4 to 6 hours), *acetaminophen* (1000 mg twice a day), or both, are used for postinjection soreness.
5.   Movement of the toes must be *restricted* for 3 to 4 weeks by limiting all unnecessary walking and standing.
6.   Recommend shortening the stride: Tell the patient to take extra time when walking to and from work.
7.   *Injection* can be repeated at 6 weeks with corticosteroid if pain recurs or persists.
8.   Request plain film radiographs of the foot and a *consultation* with a surgical orthopedist or podiatrist if two consecutive injections fail to control pain and the patient is willing to undergo an operation that may result in permanent numbness.

OUTCOME AND FURTHER WORK-UP: Local corticosteroid injection provides excellent long-term control of symptoms when combined with general foot care. The triamcinolone injectables are effective in reducing the perineural inflammation and fibrosis around the nerve. Because the reduction of the perineural fibrosis is gradual, the condition should be observed for at least 2 months before proceeding to surgery. Refractory cases should be referred to podiatry or orthopedics for definitive neurectomy.

APPENDIX

SUMMARY OF PHYSICAL THERAPY EXERCISES
RADIOLOGY AND PROCEDURES
SUPPORTS, BRACES, AND CASTS
NONSTEROIDAL ANTI-INFLAMMATORY DRUGS
CORTICOSTEROIDS
CALCIUM SUPPLEMENTATION
LABORATORY TESTS IN RHEUMATOLOGY
SYNOVIAL FLUID ANALYSIS
REFERENCES

SUMMARY OF PHYSICAL THERAPY EXERCISES

These are the physical therapy treatments and exercises used in recovery, rehabilitation, and the prevention of the most common musculoskeletal conditions. They are listed in the sequence that ensures maximum patient compliance (focusing on simplicity) and optimal outcome (see the individual diagnosis for the exact timing of these exercises relative to radiographic studies, corticosteroid injection, etc.). The most commonly prescribed **stretching exercises** used to restore range of motion are listed. In order to restore muscular support and tendon integrity, emphasis is placed on the **isometric toning exercises** rather than **active exercises** that combine toning and movement. In general, patients are much more likely to tolerate the isometric toning exercises early in the recovery phase because they do not require joint movement. The active exercises should be delayed until the patient has restored range of motion and muscle tone and tendon integrity isometrically.

CERVICAL STRAIN: Trapezial and cervical muscle stretching exercises in rotation, lateral bending, and flexion; heat and massage; ultrasound; gentle cervical traction beginning at 5 pounds for 5 minutes and gradually increasing to 15 pounds for 10 minutes twice a day

CERVICAL RADICULOPATHY: As with cervical strain with greater emphasis on traction (note that traction may aggravate the radicular symptoms of a herniated disk)

GREATER OCCIPITAL NEURITIS: Ice applications; trapezial and cervical muscle stretching exercises in rotation, lateral bending, and flexion

TEMPOROMANDIBULAR JOINT ARTHRITIS: Ice applications; gentle stretching of the muscles of mastication by opening and closing the jaw

IMPINGEMENT SYNDROME: Ice for acute symptoms; the weighted pendulum stretching exercise begun as a dangle without motion and then gradually adding circular motion as tolerated; isometric toning exercises of external and internal rotation

ROTATOR CUFF TENDINITIS: Ice over the lateral shoulder for acute symptoms; the weighted pendulum stretching exercise begun as a dangle without motion and then gradually adding circular motion as tolerated; isometric toning of abduction and external rotation (but only after the acute symptoms have resolved)

FROZEN SHOULDER: Heat over the shoulder; the weighted pendulum stretching exercise; passive stretching in abduction, external rotation, or both, depending on which direction has been affected the most; isometric toning exercises of abduction and external rotation (but only after the range of motion has significantly improved)

SUBSCAPULARIS BURSITIS: Ice over the upper back; isometric toning of the adduction and internal rotation

GLENOHUMERAL OSTEOARTHRITIS: Ice over the anterior shoulder; the weighted pendulum stretching exercise with modest added weight (2 to 5 pounds); isometric toning of external and internal rotation to enhance the stability of the joint

MULTIDIRECTIONAL INSTABILITY: Isometric toning of external and internal rotation followed by general muscle-toning exercises of the posterior deltoid, trapezius, and biceps

ROTATOR CUFF TENDON TEAR: Heat over the shoulder; the weighted pendulum stretching exercise; isometric toning of the abduction and external rotation (performed very gradually, just to the edge of discomfort and no further)

ACROMIOCLAVICULAR SPRAIN: Ice; general shoulder conditioning

BICIPITAL TENDINITIS: Ice over the anterior humeral head; phonophoresis; weighted pendulum stretching exercise; isometric toning of the elbow flexors

LATERAL EPICONDYLITIS: Ice over the lateral epicondyle; phonophoresis; isometric toning of gripping; isometric toning of wrist extension (only after grip has been restored)

OLECRANON BURSITIS: Ice

RADIOHUMERAL JOINT: Ice over the lateral joint; gentle passive stretching exercises in flexion and extension

DORSAL GANGLION OF THE WRIST: Isometric toning of the wrist in flexion and extension indicated when significant underlying wrist arthritis is present

DE QUERVAIN'S TENOSYNOVITIS: Ice over the radial styloid; phonophoresis; gentle stretching exercises of the thumb in flexion

CARPOMETACARPAL ARTHRITIS: Ice over the base of the thumb; phonophoresis; isometric toning of thumb extension and abduction

CARPAL TUNNEL SYNDROME: Ergonomic adjustments at the work station; passive stretching exercises of the finger flexors; manual stretching of the transverse carpal ligament

RADIOCARPAL JOINT: Ice over the dorsum; passive range of motion exercises in flexion and extension; isometric toning of the wrist in flexion and extension

METATARSOPHALANGEAL JOINT: Ice over the dorsum of the hand; gentle passive range of motion exercises in flexion and extension

TRIGGER FINGER: Passive stretching exercises in extension

TENDON CYSTS: None

DUPUYTREN'S CONTRACTURE: Heat the palm; lanolin cream massage of the palmar nodules; passive stretching exercises in extension

OSTEOARTHRITIS OF THE HAND: Heat paraffin wax dipping using a Crock-Pot; gentle passive range of motion exercises in extension and flexion

RHEUMATOID ARTHRITIS: Heat paraffin wax dipping using a Crock-Pot; gentle passive stretching exercises to preserve range of motion; occupational aids

COSTOCHONDRITIS: Ice directly over the rib; phonophoresis of a hydrocortisone gel is of questionable value

STERNOCLAVICULAR JOINT: Ice directly over the joint; phonophoresis of a hydrocortisone gel is of questionable value; general shoulder conditioning

LUMBOSACRAL STRAIN: Ice alternating with heat; aerobic exercises; William's flexion exercises of the erector spinae, gluteus maximus, and the flank muscles (knee-chest pulls, pelvic rocks, and side bends); active toning of the erector spinae muscles (weighted side-bend exercises, modified sit-ups, or equipment); lumbar traction or vertical stretching exercises

LUMBOSACRAL RADICULOPATHY: As for lumbosacral strain with cautious stretching and toning only after the acute radicular symptoms have significantly improved; a transcutaneous electrical nerve stimulation (TENS) unit for chronic pain

SACROILIAC JOINT: Ice alternating with heat; aerobic exercises; stretching exercises of the erector spinae, gluteus maximus, and the flank muscles (knee-chest pulls, pelvic rocks, and side bends); active toning of the erector spinae muscles (weighted side-bend exercises, modified sit-ups, or equipment)

COCCYGODYNIA: Toning of gluteus maximum with active leg extension exercises

TROCHANTERIC BURSITIS: Heat; cross-leg stretching exercise for gluteus medius; knee-chest pulls for gluteus maximus; ultrasound; a TENS unit for the chronic case

GLUTEUS MEDIUS BURSITIS: As for trochanteric bursitis

OSTEOARTHRITIS OF THE HIP: Passive stretching exercises for the adductors, rotators, and glutei (knee-chest pulls, figure-of-four stretches, sitting cross-legged style); toning exercises of the iliopsoas and glutei (straight-leg-raise and leg-extension exercises)

MERALGIA PARESTHETICA: Abdominal muscle toning (weighted side bends, modified sit-ups, crunches, etc.)

PATELLOFEMORAL DISEASES: Ice over the anterior knee; straight-leg-raise exercise and leg extensions to tone the quadriceps and hamstring muscles; cautious use of exercise equipment (limiting flexion to no greater than 30 to 45 degrees)

KNEE EFFUSION: Ice and elevation plus crutches for acute symptoms; the straight-leg-raise and leg-extension exercises for muscle toning; active exercises with caution

OSTEOARTHRITIS OF THE KNEE: As for knee effusion

PREPATELLAR BURSITIS: Ice over the bursa; quadriceps and hamstring toning play a minor role

ANSERINE BURSITIS: Ice over the medial tibial plateau; phonophoresis; general toning of the quadriceps and hamstring muscles (straight-leg-raise exercise, exercise equipment, etc.)

BAKER'S CYST: As for knee effusion

MEDIAL COLLATERAL LIGAMENT SPRAIN: Ice over the medial tibial plateau; straight-leg-raise exercises without weights; straight-leg-raise and leg-extension exercises with weights; cautious use of exercise equipment (limiting flexion to no greater than 30 degrees)

MEDIAL MENISCAL TEAR: As for knee effusion with greater emphasis on toning exercises

ANKLE SPRAIN: Ice over the lateral ankle and elevation; gentle, passive range of motion exercises in dorsiflexion and extension followed by inversion and eversion; isometric toning of posterior tibialis, peroneus, and anterior tibialis (inversion, eversion, and dorsiflexion, respectively)

ANKLE ARTHRITIS: Ice over the anterior ankle and elevation; gentle passive range of motion exercises in dorsiflexion and plantar flexion; isometric toning of dorsiflexion and plantar flexion

ACHILLES TENDINITIS: Ice over the swollen tendon; phonophoresis; passive stretching in dorsiflexion (the wall stretching exercise) followed by more active stretching; isometric toning of the tendon in plantar flexion

PRE-ACHILLES BURSITIS: Ice over the heel; passive and active stretching exercises of the Achilles tendon in dorsiflexion

RETROCALCANEAL BURSITIS: As for pre-Achilles bursitis

POSTERIOR TIBIALIS TENOSYNOVITIS: Ice over the medial ankle acutely; gentle, passive stretching exercises in dorsiflexion and eversion

PLANTAR FASCIITIS: Ice over the plantar heel; massage at the origin of the fascia on the calcaneus; active Achilles tendon stretching in dorsiflexion

HEEL PAD SYNDROME: Ice over the plantar heel; massage over the bottom of the heel

BUNIONS: Ice and elevation; passive stretching exercises of dorsiflexion and plantar flexion

ADVENTITIAL BURSITIS OF THE FIRST METATARSOPHALANGEAL JOINT: Ice and elevation; passive stretching exercises of dorsiflexion and plantar flexion

GOUT: Ice and elevation

HAMMER TOES: Heat; passive and active stretching exercises of the extensor tendons (in plantar flexion)

MORTON'S NEUROMA: None

Table 1 Radiology and Procedures

Procedure	Findings—Significance
Neck	
Cervical spine series (lateral, PA, oblique)	"Reversed or straightened curve"—cervical or upper back muscle spasm Localized straightening of the cervical curve—local muscle spasm from a herniated disk Facet joint and vertebral body spurring and sclerosis—cervical osteoarthritis Subluxation of two vertebral bodies—spondylolisthesis or fracture Large anterior osteophytes causing "a lump in the throat"; "dumbbell"-shaped foraminal encroachment from cervical radiculopathy (>50% narrowing)
Flexion and extension	Odontoid subluxation from rheumatoid disease (nl views of the neck 3.5 mm odontoid to atlas)
MRI of the cervical spine (75% ordered for radiculopathy and 20% for myelopathy)	Common findings: herniated disk, foraminal encroachment disease, bony pathology such as osteomyelitis, metastases, etc., and intrinsic disease of the spinal cord
EMG of the upper extremity	Denervation associated with nerve root compression (used in the evaluation of poorly defined arm pains)
Shoulder	
PA, external rotation and Y-outlet view	Calcification—rotator cuff or bicipital tendinitis Greater tubercle sclerosis and erosion—subacromial impingement Superior migration of the humeral head—rotator cuff tendon tear AC joint width >4-5 mm—second-degree AC separation clavicle superior to the acromion—third degree AC separation Squared-off ends of the acromion and clavicle, narrowing of the joint, sclerosis, and bone spurring—AC joint osteoarthritis Anterior or posterior position of the humerus—dislocation Bony pathology
Axillary view	Glenohumeral joint narrowing, sclerosis, spur formation are characteristics of glenohumeral osteoarthritis (the best view for measuring the glenohumeral joint space)
Acromial arch view	Narrowing, irregularity of the acromion or AC joint spur encroachment—subacromial impingement
Weighted views of the AC joint	AC joint space >4-5 mm—second-degree AC shoulder separation

Arthrography with or without CT	Contracted glenohumeral space—frozen shoulder dye leaking into the subacromial bursa—rotator cuff tendon tear irregularities of the glenohumeral joint—osteoarthritis or rheumatoid disease
	Irregularity of the glenoid labrum—labral tear
MRI scanning	Separation/irregularity of the rotator cuff tendon—"tear"
Subacromial lidocaine injection test for rotator cuff tendinitis	75% pain relief and >75% of external rotation and abduction strength—uncomplicated rotator cuff tendinitis
	Poor pain relief, <75% strength—rotator cuff tendon tear

Elbow

PA and lateral	Triceps calcification—incidental finding
	Radial head and ulnar osteophytes, joint space narrowing, sclerosis—osteoarthritis
MRI scanning	Irregularity of the articular cartilage— osteochondritis dissecans with or without loose bodies
NCV of the ulnar nerve	Slowing—cubital tunnel syndrome
Bursal aspiration	Crystals—gout or pseudogout
	Gram-positive cocci—*Staphylococcus aureus*
	Bloody or serous effusion—traumatic bursitis

Wrist

PA, lateral, and oblique	Radiocarpal joint space narrowing, sclerosis of the radius, irregular shape to the navicular, and increased gap between the navicular and the lunate—radiocarpal osteoarthritis
	Sclerosis of the navicular—avascular necrosis of the navicular
	Sclerosis of the lunate—avascular necrosis of the lunate or Kienbock's disease
	Calcification of the triangular cartilage— pseudogout
	Abnormal alignment of the carpal bones— subluxation of the navicular or lunate, etc.
	Increased gap between the lunate and navicular— subluxation, carpal dissociation
	Loss of the uniform 1 mm spacing between the carpal bones—RA or osteoarthritis
Coned-down view of the navicular	Cortical irregularities or fracture line—navicular fracture
Carpal tunnel view	
NCV of the median nerve	Slowing of the nerve—carpal tunnel (30% false negative!)
	Subluxation of the lunate causing CTS

Thumb
PA, lateral, and oblique

Sclerosis, narrowing, spurring, and subluxation of the carpometacarpal joint—CMC osteoarthritis

Asymmetrical narrowing, sclerosis, spurring of the MP joint—osteoarthritis

Hand
PA, lateral, and oblique

Asymmetrical joint space narrowing, osteophytes, and ("soft tissue technique") bony sclerosis of the DIP or PIP joints—osteoarthritis

Punctate calcification in the soft tissues of the MCP joints—foreign body reaction to gravel, corticosteroid injection, etc.

Juxta-articular osteoporosis of the MCP or PIP joints—early RA

Symmetrical joint space narrowing and periarticular erosions—advanced RA

Asymmetrical erosive change of the proximal phalangeal joint without juxta-articular osteoporosis or dramatic joint space narrowing—chronic tophaceous gout

Fluffy periosteal elevation of the proximal phalanges—correlation with sausage digit of Reiter's disease

"Pencil-and-cup" deformity of destructive arthritis—psoriasis

Unilateral juxta-articular osteoporosis—Sudeck's atrophy of bone; reflex sympathetic dystrophy

Lumbosacral Spine
PA and lateral

Loss of the normal lumbar lordosis—paraspinal muscle spasm

Sclerosis and narrowing of the facet joints—osteoarthritis; spinal stenosis

Wedge-shaped vertebral body—compression fracture

S-shaped curve—scoliosis

S-shaped curve with rotation—rotatory scoliosis

Anterior displacement of one vertebral body over another—spondylolisthesis

Bony pathology

Oblique views

Missing pars intra-articularis (the neck of the Scottie dog)—spondylosis of spondylolisthesis

Flexion and extension

Increased movement of the vertebral bodies—views spondylolisthesis instability

MRI scanning

As for CT scanning with greater detail of nerve and cord integrity and of postoperative cases with scar tissue

CT scanning (many indications and uses—75% for radiculopathy, 20% for metastatic work-up, 5% for advanced arthritis)

Bulging disk compressing the spinal nerve, lateral recess narrowing, fragmented disk lodged in the lateral recess—radiculopathy

Narrowing of the spinal canal—spinal stenosis

Bony pathology

Bone scanning	Increased uptake is nonspecific in osteoarthritis, bony pathology, osteomyelitis, etc.
Myelography	Replaced by CT and MRI

Hip

PA and lateral (order standing PA of both hips on 1 cassette)	Joint space narrowing between the superior acetabulum and femoral head, bony sclerosis and a variable degree of superior acetabular osteophytes—osteoarthritis
	Migration of the femoral head into the pelvis—"protrusio acetabulae"
	Sclerotic line and "step off" at proximal third of the head of the femur—avascular necrosis (late)
	Calcification over the lateral femur—trochanteric or gluteus medius bursa (uncommon)
	Various bony abnormalities
Frog leg view	Alternate view of femoral head
Standing AP pelvis with level	Measurement of leg length discrepancy
	Widening and irregularity of the symphysis pubis—osteitis pubis or diastasis
Oblique views of the pelvis	Bony sclerosis of the sacrum and ileum, bony erosions, widening of the joint—sacroiliitis
	Bony sclerosis of the iliac side of the SI joint—osteitis condensans ilii (benign)
Lateral views of the coccyx	Abnormal anterior angulation of the coccyx—post-traumatic coccygodynia
Bone scanning—avascular necrosis or various bony abnormalities	Diffuse uptake—arthritis, infection
	Uptake in the proximal third of the femoral head
MRI scanning	Irregularity of the proximal third of the femoral head—avascular necrosis (90% of all hip MRI)

Knee

PA and lateral (order bilateral standing lateral PA on 1 cassette)	Medial joint space narrowing (nl 1 mm wider than the lateral)—early osteoarthritis
	Asymmetrical narrowing, increased tibial sclerosis, and tibial or femoral osteophytes—advanced osteoarthritis
	Narrowing of the medial joint space, valgus angle of the knee <9 degrees—osteoarthritis
	Meniscal calcification—chondrocalcinosis
	Osteochondritis dissecans
	Linear calcification of the MCL
	Pellagrina steida syndrome (old MCL injury)
	Various bony abnormalities
	Calcification in the joint—loose body
	Calcification outside the joint—flabella
Merchant view of the patella ("sunrise" view)	Patella does not sit in the center of the patellar femoral groove—subluxation or frank dislocation
	Asymmetrical joint space narrowing, patellar sclerosis and patellar pole osteophytes—patellofemoral osteoarthritis

Tunnel view	Well-circumscribed calcified body between the femoral condyles—loose body
MRI scanning of the knee	Irregularities of the menisci—tears, congenital defects, etc.
	Irregularities of the articular cartilage—arthritis, osteochondritis dissecans, etc.
	Disrupted cruciate ligaments—torn anterior or posterior cruciate
Arthrography	Supplanted by MRI
Ultrasound	Popliteal mass—Baker's cyst or popliteal artery aneurysm
Bursa aspiration	Crystals—gout, pseudogout
	Gram-positive cocci—*S. aureus*
	Serous or bloody aspirate—traumatic bursitis
Arthroscopy, diagnostic	For confirming meniscal, patellar, or cruciate pathology seen on MRI scanning

Ankle and Lower Leg

PA, lateral, and "mortis" (many indications and uses)	Joint space narrowing, sclerosis, and hypertrophic views osteophytes—tibiotalar arthritis
	Calcification of the Achilles tendon—nearly always asymptomatic
	Calcification posterior to the Achilles tendon insertion—pre-Achilles bursitis
	Calcaneal heel spur—possible plantar fasciitis
	Fleck of calcium off the proximal fifth metatarsal—avulsion fracture of peroneus longus—severe ankle sprain
	Well-circumscribed calcified bodies adjacent to the tarsal bones—sesamoid bones that are rarely symptomatic
	Talar bone irregularities in the severely sprained ankle—lateral process fracture of the dome of the talus, posterior process fracture, and others
Varus stress radiograph	Talus shift and subluxation with stress—chronic lateral instability of the ankle
Oblique views of the ankle	Tarsal bone fusion—tarsal coalition
NCV of the posterior tibialis nerve	Slowing of nerve transmission—tarsal tunnel syndrome

Foot

PA, lateral, and oblique	The first MTP joint, sclerosis and asymmetrical narrowing—bunions
	Abnormal angulation of the MTP and PIP joints—hammer toes
	Juxta-articular osteoporosis of the MTP and PIP joints—rheumatoid arthritis
	Thickened cortex of the third or fourth metatarsal shafts—stress fracture
	Hypertrophic spurring at the first metatarsal first cuneiform—the dorsal bunion

199

	Calcification of the posterior third of the calcaneus—calcaneal stress fracture
	Diffuse osteoporosis of the bones of the foot—reflex sympathetic dystrophy
	Bony erosion with an "overhanging margin"—gout
Standing lateral foot	Flattening of the longitudinal arch (pes planus) vs. high arch (pes cavus)
Sesamoid view of the big toe	Irregularities of the sesamoid bones—bibartite sesamoid bone vs. fracture

AC, acromioclavicular; CT, computed tomography; CMC, carpometacarpal; CTS, carpal tunnel syndrome; DIP, distal interphalangeal; EMG, electromyography; MCL, medial collateral ligament; MCP, metacarpophalangeal; MRI, magnetic resonance imaging; MTP, metatarsophalangeal; NCV, nerve conduction velocity; nl, normal; PA, posteroanterior; PIP, proximal interphalangeal; RA, rheumatoid arthritis; SI, sacroiliac.

Table 2 Supports, Braces, and Casts

	COST ($)
Neck	
Soft cervical collar	8-9
Philadelphia collar	
Soft	35-40
Hard	60-65
Water bag cervical traction unit	25-40
Shoulder	
Simple shoulder sling	4-7
Hanging cast	65-70
Clavicular strap	10-12
Shoulder immobilizer	19-20
Universal	19-20
Velcro	31-32
Abduction pillow	50-52
Elbow	
Tennis elbow band	5-12
Neoprene pull-on elbow brace	10-12
Wrist	
Simple Velcro wrist support	6-7
Velcro wrist immobilizer with metal stays	17-18
Short-arm cast	
Plaster	25-27
Fiberglass	45-47
Sugar tong splint	
Plaster	30-32
Fiberglass	65-70
Radial gutter splint	
Plaster	21-23
Fiberglass	39-42
Dorsal hood splint	
Plaster	15-16
Fiberglass	28-30
Ulnar gutter splint	
Plaster	21-23
Fiberglass	39-42
Thumb	
Taping the CMC joint	1-2
Padded shell Velcro thumb splint	26-28
Thermoplastic molded thumb splint	25-26

Thumb (cont.)

Thumb spica cast
Plaster	28-30
Fiberglass	52-54

Finger

Buddy-taping	1-2
Tube splint	15-16
Stax splint	3-4
Dorsal splint	2-3
Metal finger splint	3-4
Silicone squeeze ball or grip putty	3-4
Spring-loaded metal gripper	10-11

Lumbosacral Spine

Neoprene waist wrap	10-15
Velcro LS corset	25-32
Elastic sacroiliac belt	12-14
LS elastic binder with heated plastic shield	125
Sacroiliac support, corset type	45-50
Three-point extension brace	260-270

Hip

Crutches	21-25

Knee

Ace wrap	3-4
Neoprene pull-on knee brace	
Simple	7-8
Patellar cut-out	16-17
Velcro kneepads	15-20
Patellar strap	15-16
Velcro patellar restraining immobilizer	35-36
Velcro straight-leg brace	
18 inches	36-38
24 inches	44-46
Metal-hinged braces	
Lennox-Hill	800-900
Off-loader brace	800-900

Ankle

Neoprene pull-on ankle brace	7-8
New-Skin or moleskin	2-3
Velcro ankle brace	29-30
Stirrup brace	35-40
T-brace	30-32
Rocker-bottom plastic ankle immobilizer	45-56

Ankle (cont.)

Short-leg walking cast	
Plaster	51-54
Fiberglass	94-100
Unna boot	21-22
Athletic taping of the ankle	4-5
Ankle foot orthosis	15-60

Foot

Heel cushion	3-5
Heel cups	5-8
Padded insoles	8-12
Padded insoles with arch supports	20-24
Plastic orthotic arch supports	
Over the counter	25-27
Custom made, plaster molded	75-80
Bunion shield	4-5
Metatarsal bar	20-25
Hammer toe crest	14-16
Metatarsal pad	4-5
Felt rings (for corns and calluses)	2-3
Pumice stone	2-3
Rubber toe spacer	3-4

CMC, carpometacarpal; LS, lumbosacral.

NONSTEROIDAL ANTI-INFLAMMATORY DRUGS

The effectiveness of the oral nonsteroidal anti-inflammatory drugs (NSAIDs) in controlling the body's inflammatory response to irritation and injury depends on (1) the length of time of administration, (2) the penetration of the drug into the joint or inflamed tissue, and (3) the degree of local inflammation. To maximize the clinical response, these medications must be taken in full dose for a minimum of 10 to 14 days. The anti-inflammatory effect peaks at 7 to 10 days as opposed to the analgesic or antipyretic effect, which occurs within 24 to 48 hours. If the inflammatory signs and symptoms have abated, the dosage should be tapered gradually over the ensuing 1 to 2 weeks. In general, the inflammatory response must be suppressed for 3 to 4 weeks to allow the body to repair the injured joint or soft tissue.

Tissue penetration is the second most important factor determining the effectiveness of NSAIDs. This is the likely explanation why the conditions affecting the large joints have a much more predictable response to these drugs than conditions affecting the medium and small joints. The conditions that affect the shoulder, hip, and knee, such as rotator cuff tendinitis, trochanteric bursitis of the hip, and osteoarthritis of the knee, commonly respond to the NSAIDs. By contrast, lateral epicondylitis, trigger finger, and plantar fasciitis, the conditions affecting the medium and small joints of the body, respond poorly. It is for this reason that the conditions affecting the wrist, hands, ankles and feet are best treated with immobilization, local injection, or both rather than with NSAIDs.

Not all conditions affecting the skeleton develop a measurable inflammatory response. Bony fractures rarely develop a significant inflammation. Certain musculoskeletal conditions are purely mechanical in nature with little secondary inflammation such as meniscal tear of the knee or the reactive muscle spasm of the neck, low back strain, and so forth. This is not to say these drugs should not be used at all for these conditions. NSAIDs provide good pain control and are an excellent substitute for narcotic analgesics.

NSAIDs are contraindicated in patients diagnosed with active ulcer disease, uncontrolled reflux, bleeding disorders, or active renal disease, patients treated with warfarin (Coumadin), and patients who have suffered allergic reactions to the drugs. NSAIDs must be used with caution in diabetics with renal disease, patients with poorly controlled blood pressure, and patients with advanced congestive heart failure.

Table 3 Nonsteroidal Anti-inflammatory Drugs

Generic	Trade	Dose (Max Daily)	Cost per 100 in Dollars
Acetaminophen	Tylenol ES	1000 (4 g)	3-5
Salicylate			
Acetylsalicylic acid*	Anacin, Ascriptin, Bufferin, Ecotrin	325, 500 (5-6 g)	4-5
Choline, Mg*	Trilisate	0.5, 0.75, 1 g (3 g)	80-100
Diflunisal*	Dolobid	50, 500 (1500)	95-117
Salsalate*	Disalcid	500, 750 (3000)	25-30
Fenamates			
Meclofenamate Na*	Meclomen	50, 100 (400)	35-45
Oxicams			
Piroxicam	Feldene	10, 20 (20)	54-60
Pyrrolopyrrole			
Ketorolac tromethamine	Toradol	15, 30, 60 (120-150)	117-120
Propionic Acids			
Fenoprofen Ca*	Nalfon	200, 300, 600 (3200)	57-87
Flurbiprofen*	Ansaid	50, 100 (300)	83-124
Ibuprofen*	Advil, Motrin, Nuprin, Rufen	200, 400, 600, 800 (3000)	15-18
Ketoprofen*	Orudis	25, 50, 75 (300)	90-120
Naproxen*	Naprosyn	250, 375, 500 (1500)	35-45
Naproxen Na	Anaprox	275, 550 (1650)	100-141
Acetic Acids			
Diclofenac Na*	Voltaren	25, 50, 75 (200)	54-116
Indomethacin*	Indomethacin	25, 50, 75SR (200)	20-32
Nabumetone*	Relafen	500, 750 (2000)	99-120
Sulindac*	Clinoril	150. 200 (400)	35-45
Tolmetin Na*	Tolectin	200, 400 (1800)	22-61
Pyranocarboxylic acid			
Etodolac	Lodine	200, 300 (1200)	73-84
COX-2 Inhibitors			
Celecoxib	Celebrex	100, 200 (200)	198-316
Rofecoxib	Vioxx	12.5, 25 (50)	250-331
Valdecoxib	Bextra	10	300-360

*Older NSAIDs are generally only available in generic form. COX-2, cyclooxyenase-2.

Table 4 Corticosteroids

Corticosteroid (abbr) (Generic)	Strength (in mg/mL)	Equivalent mg of Hydrocortisone
Short-Acting Preparations ("Soluble")		
Hydrocortone Phosphate (H) (hydrocortone sodium phosphate)	25, 50	25, 50
Hydeltrasol (H20) (prednisolone sodium phosphate)	20	80
Long-Acting Preparations (Depot or Time Released)		
Kenalog (K40) (triamcinolone acetonide)	40	200
Aristospan (A20) (triamcinolone hexacetonide)	20	100
Depo-Medrol (D80) (methylprednisolone acetate)	20, 40, 80	100-300
Decadron Phosphate (Dex8) (dexamethasone sodium phosphate)	4, 8	100, 200
Hydeltra-T.B.A. (HTBA) (prednisolone tebutate)	20	80
Combination Preparations (Both Soluble and Depot)		
Celestone Soluspan (C6) (betamethasone)	6	150

Table 5 Calcium Supplementation

	Amount of or Tablet Size	Calcium Content (in mg)	Yearly Cost ($)
Foods			
Milk (nonfat)	1 cup	290-300	200
Yogurt	1 cup	240-400	950
Cheese slice	1 oz	160-260	260
Cottage cheese	½ cup	80-100	960
Broccoli	1 cup	160-180	2000
Tofu	4 oz	145-155	1500
Salmon, canned	3 oz	170-200	3700
Supplements			
Calcium carbonate			
Oyster shell (generic)	625, 1250, 1500	250, 500, 600	40
Os-Cal	625, 1250	250, 500	108
Os-Cal + D	625, 1250	250, 500	107
Tums E-X	750	300	55
Calcium Rich Rolaids	550	220	53
Caltrate	1500	600	108
Caltrate + D (125 international units)	1500	600	108
Calcium phosphate			
Posture	1565	600	115
Posture D (125 international units)	1565	600	115
Calcium lactate	650	85	350
Calcium gluconate 9	975	90	522
Calcium citrate			
Citracal 950	950	200	162
Citracal 1500+			
(200 international units)	1500	315	162

LABORATORY TESTS IN RHEUMATOLOGY

Rheumatoid Factor

"The most significant laboratory abnormality in rheumatoid arthritis!"

Antibodies to the Fc portion of IgG

May take 6 months to become positive (it is *insensitive* as a screening test)

75%-80% of adults with RA have significant titers, i.e., >1:160, and 20%-25% are seronegative; only 20% of children with JRA are seropositive—seropositivity correlates with HLA-DR4 haplotype

IgM rheumatoid factor is most common

High titers are associated with more severe disease, active joint disease, presence of nodules, and poorer prognosis

IgG rheumatoid factor is associated with more severe disease

IgA rheumatoid factor is associated with bony erosions

Positive RF can occur in normal individuals, TB, bacterial endocarditis, syphilis, pulmonary fibrosis, chronic active hepatitis, infectious hepatitis, as well as Sjögren's, SLE, PSS, and polymyositis—there are many false positives!

Crystals

Best identified using a polarizing microscope

Monosodium urate crystals—needle shaped, negatively birefringent, gout

Calcium pyrophosphate dihydrate crystals—polygonal, positive birefringent, pseudogout

Calcium hydroxyapatite crystals—glossy globules that stain with alizarin red S stain on light microscopy, electron microscopy for specific chemical content, calcium hydroxyapatite crystal deposition disease

Antinuclear Antibodies
ANA

Homogeneous—reacts against deoxynucleoprotein and histone DNA; the **most common** pattern of ANA; least specific for SLE (many false positives)

Rimmed or membranous—reacts against double-stranded DNA and native DNA; uncommon; far more specific for SLE than homogeneous

Speckled—reacts against extractable nuclear antigens (ENAs); 30% of patients with SLE

Nucleolar—reacts against ribonucleoprotein (RNP); unusual pattern; more suggestive of PSS than SLE

Centromeric—reacts against topoisomerase I; two thirds of CREST syndrome

DNA

Anti-DNA—reacts against double-stranded DNA; diagnostic of SLE; correlates with disease activity in most patients

ENA

Anti-RNP—reacts against antigen susceptible to RNase digestion; 50% of SLE and all patients with mixed connective tissue disease

Anti-Sm—also called anti-Smith; the only ENA that is specific for SLE; only 15%-30% of SLE (low sensitivity)

Anti-Ro—also called anti-SSA; reacts against RNA-protein antigen; 25%-40% of SLE patients; 70% of Sjögren's syndrome patients

Anti-La—also called anti-SSB; reacts against RNA-protein antigen; 10%-15% of SLE patients; 50% of Sjögren's syndrome patients

Interpretation

The testing for autoantibodies (ANA testing) should *not* be used as a screen for rheumatic disease! The ANA test should be used to confirm the clinical diagnosis of a patient with symptoms compatible with SLE!

Positive ANA: Consider the clinical setting; titers <1:160 with few clinical criteria for SLE are probably false positives. Moderate titers between 1:320 and 1:5120 deserve further evaluation (a high titer is greater than 1:5120); moderate or high titers deserve anti-DNA and anti-ENA testing for confirmation of SLE or other rheumatic conditions

Positive ANA from drugs: often a homogeneous pattern; procainamide, hydralazine, and isoniazid

Positive ANA and diseases: common in patients older than age 50 with chronic inflammatory conditions such as active hepatitis, pulmonary fibrosis, infections, and malignancy, particularly lymphoma; usually the titers are <1:640

Positive ANA with age: 5%-10% of 50-year-olds have a positive ANA; 20% of 70-year-olds have a positive ANA

Clinical Criteria for SLE

Malar rash; discoid rash; photosensitivity; oral ulcers; arthritis; serositis; renal disease of proteinuria and cellular casts; neurologic disorders of seizures or psychosis; hematologic disorders of hemolytic anemia or leukopenia or lymphopenia or thrombocytopenia; positive LE prep, anti-DNA, anti-Sm, or false-positive VDRL; and positive ANA

ANA, antinuclear antibody; CREST, calcinosis cutis, Raynaud's phenomenon, esophageal dysfunction, sclerodactyly, and telangiectasia; DNA, deoxyribonucleic acid; IgA, immunoglobulin A; IgG, immunoglobulin G; IgM, immunoglobulin M; JRA, juvenile rheumatoid arthritis; LE, lupus erythematosus; PSS, progressive systemic sclerosis; RA, rheumatoid arthritis; RF, rheumatoid factor; RNase, ribonuclease; SLE, systemic lupus erythematosus; TB, tuberculosis; VDRL, Venereal Disease Research Laboratory.

Table 6 Synovial Fluid Analysis

	Normal Synovial Fluid	Noninflammatory Fluid (Group 1)	Inflammatory Fluid (Group 2)	Infectious Fluid (Group 3)
Appearance	Clear	Clear or Sl turbid Bloody	Turbid	Very turbid
Color	Colorless or Sl yellow	Yellow	Yellow-white	White-yellow
Viscosity	Normal	Decreased	Decreased	Decreased
Total WBCs per mm^3	<200	<2500	2500-25,000	> 50,000
Differential (% Polys)	7%	13%-20%	50%-70%	90%
Blood vs. fluid glucose difference (mg/dL)	0	5	0-30	70-90
Clinical examples	Osteoarthritis Patellofemoral syndrome Mechanical derangement SLE Hyperparathyroid	Rheumatoid arthritis Pseudogout Gout Reiter's syndrome GC Rheumatic fever TB SLE	Septic arthritis TB	

GC, gonorrhea; Sl, slightly; SLE, systemic lupus erythematosus; TB, tuberculosis; WBCs, white blood cells.

REFERENCES

History

Hollander JL, Brown EM, Jessar RA, Brown CY. Hydrocortisone and cortisone injected into arthritic joints: comparative effects of and use of hydrocortisone as a local antiarthritic. JAMA 147:1929-1635, 1951.

Lapidus PW, Guidotti FP. Local injections of hydrocortisone in 495 orthopedic patients. Industr Med Surg 6:234-244, 1957.

Technique

Ellis RM, Hollingworth GR, MacCollum MS. Comparison of injection techniques for shoulder pain: results of a double-blind, randomized study. BMJ 287:1339-1341, 1983.

Use

Anderson BC. Office Orthopedics for Primary Care, 1st ed. Philadelphia, WB Saunders, 1995.

Anderson BC, Kaye S. Treatment of flexor tenosynovitis of the hand ("trigger finger") with corticosteroids. Arch Intern Med 151:153-156, 1991.

Anderson BC, Manthey R, Brouns MC. Treatment of DeQuervain's tenosynovitis with corticosteroids. Arthritis Rheum 34:793-798, 1991.

Balch HW, Gibson JM, El Ghorbarey AF, et al. Repeated corticosteroid injections into knee joints. Rheumatol Rehab 19:62-66, 1970.

Barber FA, Sutker AN. Iliotibial band syndrome. Sports Med 14:144-148, 1992.

Boyd HB, McLeod AC. Tennis elbow. J Bone Joint Surg 55A:1183-1197, 1973.

Brooker AF Jr. The surgical approach to refractory trochanteric bursitis. Johns Hopkins Med J 145:98-100, 1979.

Day BH, Govindasamy N. Corticosteroid injections in the treatment of tennis elbow. Practitioner 220:459-462, 1978.

Ege-Rasmussen KJ, Fano N. Trochanteric bursitis. Treatment by corticosteroid injection. Scand J Rheumatol 14:417-420, 1985.

Fillion PL. Treatment of lateral epicondylitis. Am J Occup Ther 45:340-343, 1991.

Foster JB, Goodman HV. The effect of local corticosteroid injection on median nerve conduction in carpal tunnel syndrome. Ann Phys Med 6:287-294, 1962.

Gray RG, Kiem IM, Gottlieb NL. Intratendon sheath corticosteroid treatment of rheumatoid arthritis-associated and idiopathic flexor tenosynovitis. Arthritis Rheum 21:92-96, 1978.

Harvey FJ, Harvey PM, Horsly MW. De Quervain's disease: Surgical or non-surgical treatment. J Hand Surg 15A:83-87, 1990.

Hassell AB, Fowler PD, Dawes PT. Intra-bursal tetracycline in the treatment of olecranon bursitis in patients with rheumatoid arthritis. Br J Rheumatol 33:859-860, 1994.

Hill JJ, Trapp RG, Colliver JA. Survey on the use of corticosteroid injections by orthopedists. Contemp Orthop 18:39-45, 1989.

Hollander JL, Brown EM, Jessar RA, Brown CY. Hydrocortisone and cortisone injection into arthritic joints: Comparative effects of and use of hydrocortisone as a local antiarthritic agent. JAMA 147:1629-1631, 1951.

Knight JM, Thomas JC, Maurer RC. Treatment of septic olecranon and prepatellar bursitis with percutaneous placement of a suction-irrigation system. A report of 12 cases. Clin Orthop 206:90-93, 1986.

Lozman PR, Hechtman KS, Uribe JW. Combined arthroscopic management of impingement syndrome and acromioclavicular joint arthritis. J South Orthop Assoc 4:177-181, 1995.

Lyu SR. Closed division of the flexor tendon sheath for trigger finger. J Bone Joint Surg 74:418-420, 1992.

Murphy D, Failla JM, Koniuch MP. Steroid versus placebo injection for trigger finger. J Hand Surg 20:628-631, 1995.

Nakhostine M, Friedrich NF, Muller W, Kentsch A. A special high tibial osteotomy technique for treatment of unicompartmental osteoarthritis of the knee. Orthopedics 16:1255-1258, 1993.

Nirschl RP, Pettrone FA. Tennis elbow. The surgical treatment of lateral epicondylitis. J Bone Joint Surg Am 61:832-839, 1979.

Phalen GS. Carpal tunnel syndrome, 17 years of experience in diagnosis and treatment. J Bone Joint Surg 48A:211-228, 1966.

Potter HG, Hannafin JA, Morsessel RM, et al. Lateral epicondylitis: Correlation with MR imaging, surgical and histopathologic findings. Radiology 196:43-46, 1995.

Puniello MS. Iliotibial band tightness and medial patellar glide in patients with patellofemoral syndrome. J Orthop Sports Phys Ther 17:144-148, 1993.

Radanow BP, Sturzenegger M, Di Stefano G. Long term outcome after whiplash. Medicine 74:281-297, 1995.

Rothenberg RJ. Rheumatic disease aspects of leg length inequality. Semin Arthritis Rheum 17:196-205, 1988.

Shapiro S. Microsurgical carpal tunnel release. Neurosurgery 37:66-70, 1995.

Stothard J, Kumar A. A safe percutaneous procedure for trigger finger release. J R Coll Surg Edinb 39:116-117, 1994.

Weinstein DM, McCann PD, McIlveen SJ, et al. Surgical treatment of complete acromioclavicular dislocations. Am J Sports Med 23:324-331, 1995.

White RH, Paull DM, Fleming KW. Rotator cuff tendonitis: comparison of subacromial injection of a long acting corticosteroid versus oral indomethacin therapy. J Rheumatol 13:608-613, 1986.

Review
Semin Arthritis Rheum, May, 1981.

Side Effects
Bedi SS, Ellis W. Spontaneous rupture of the calcaneal tendon in rheumatoid arthritis after steroid injection. Ann Rheum Dis 29:494-495, 1970.

Hollander JL, Jessar RA, Brown EM. Intra-synovial corticosteroid therapy: a decade of use. Bull Rheum Dis 11:239-240, 1961.

Ismail AM, Balakrishnan R, Rajakumar MK. Rupture of patellar ligament after steroid infiltration, report of a case. J Bone Joint Surg 51B:503-505, 1969.

Kendall, PH. Untoward effects following local hydrocortisone injection. Ann Phys Med 4:170-175, 1961.

Kleinman M, Gross AE. Achilles tendon rupture following steroid injection. J Bone Joint Surg 65A:1345-1347, 1983.

Synovial Fluid Analysis
Cohen AS, Brandt KD, Krey PR. Synovial fluid. *In* Cohen AS (ed). Laboratory Diagnostic Procedures in the Rheumatoid Diseases, 2nd ed. Boston, Little, Brown, 1975, 1-62.

Goldenberg DL, Reed JI. Bacterial arthritis. N Engl J Med 312:764-771, 1985.

James MJ, Cleland LG, Rofe AM, Leslie AL. Intra-articular pressure and the relationship between synovial perfusion and metabolic demand. J Rheumatol 17:521-527, 1990.

Krey PR, Bailen DA. Synovial fluid leukocytosis: a study of extremes. Am J Med 67:436-442, 1979.

Ropes MW, Bauer W. Synovial Changes in Joint Disease. Cambridge, Mass, Harvard University Press, 1953.

NOTES